Emergency Cardiology

An Evidence-Based Guide to Acute Cardiac Problems

Azad Ghuran MBChB MRCP
Specialist/Research Registrar in Cardiology
Department of Cardiological Sciences
St George's Hospital Medical School
London

Neal Uren MBChB MD MRCP
Consultant Cardiologist
Department of Cardiology
Royal Infirmary of Edinburgh
Edinburgh

James Nolan MBChB MD FRCP
Consultant Cardiologist
Cardiothoracic Centre
North Staffordshire University Hospital
Stoke-on-Trent

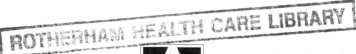

ARNOLD

A member of the Hodder Headline Group
LONDON

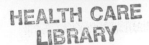
First published in Great Britain in 2003 by
Arnold, a member of the Hodder Headline Group,
338 Euston Road, London NW1 3BH

http://www.arnoldpublishers.com

Distributed in the United States of America by
Oxford University Press Inc.,
198 Madison Avenue, New York, NY10016
Oxford is a registered trademark of Oxford University Press

British Library Cataloguing in Publication Data
A catalogue record for this book is available from the British Library

Library of Congress Cataloging-in-Publication Data
A catalog record for this book is available from the Library of Congress

ISBN 0 340 80719 9

1 2 3 4 5 6 7 8 9 10

Commissioning Editor: Joanna Koster
Production Editor: Wendy Rooke
Production Controller: Bryan Eccleshall

Typeset in 9/11 Palatino by Charon Tec Pvt. Ltd, Chennai, India
Printed and bound in Spain

What do you think about this book? Or any other Arnold title?
Please send your comments to feedback.arnold@hodder.co.uk

14854

Contents

Preface

Cardiovascular disease is the most common cause of death in developed countries. Many cardiac diseases first present as an emergency in an acutely ill and unstable patient. Rapid diagnosis, assessment and intervention may alter the course and outcome in these patients, and can be lifesaving. Cardiology is unique in having a large, rapidly evolving body of clinical trial data to guide the emergency management of these patients. Consequently, this area of acute medical practice can appear highly complex, and is often a source of great stress for nursing and medical staff.

The purpose of this book is to provide concise, up-to-date evidence-based guidelines for the management of these common conditions. Each chapter provides background information on epidemiology and pathophysiology, followed by guidelines for diagnosis, treatment and the management of complications. These guidelines reflect our own evolving clinical experience, in addition to the latest advances based on recently published or presented trials. At the end of each chapter is a list of the key references which provide the evidence base for the text. Appendix C provides website addresses for useful internet sites that should help to keep readers up to date with new clinical trials and evolving management guidelines.

Appendix A provides information on intravenous drug preparation and dosing regimes, which comply with the current British National Formulary guidelines. It is important to stress that drug policies and regimes can vary or evolve with time, and you should tailor treatment regimes to local practice and to each individual patient. Appendix B provides normal ranges and formulae for commonly performed investigations.

We hope that this book will prove useful for medical and nursing staff dealing with these common problems in accident and emergency, acute medical and specialized cardiac units. The pace of change in acute cardiology is rapid, and we plan to update and improve this book on a regular basis; therefore, we would welcome feedback and comments from readers.

Producing any book is always a long and demanding process. We would like to thank the staff at Arnold for their help in producing this book, Rachel Grace for typing the manuscript and our families for supporting us during the time-consuming production of this text.

Azad Ghuran
Neal Uren
Jim Nolan

Abbreviations

ACC	American College of Cardiology
ACD	active and compression–decompression
ACE	angiotensin converting enzyme
ACT	activated clotting time
ADP	adenosine diphosphate
AF	atrial fibrillation
AHA	American Heart Association
AICD	autonomic implantable cardioverter defibrillator
aPTT	activated partial thromboplastin time
ATP	adenosine triphosphate
A-V	arteriovenous
AV	atrioventricular
AVNRT	atrioventricular nodal re-entry tachycardia
AVRT	atrioventricular re-entry tachycardia
BP	blood pressure
CABG	coronary artery bypass graft
CAD	coronary artery disease
cAMP	cyclic adenosine monophosphate
CCS	Canadian Cardiovascular Society
CCU	coronary care unit
CK	creatine kinase
CMV	cytomegalovirus
COPD	chronic obstructive pulmonary disease
CPR	cardiopulmonary resuscitation
CRP	C-reactive protein
CT	computed tomography
CTPA	computed tomography pulmonary angiography
CVA	cerebrovascular accident
DCC	direct current cardioversion
DVT	deep venous thrombosis
ECG	electrocardiogram
EF	ejection fraction
ELISA	enzyme-linked immunoadsorbent assay

EMD	electromechanical dissociation
EPS	electrophysiological study
ERC	European Resuscitation Council
ESR	erythrocyte sedimentation rate
FDP	fibrin degradation products
GI	gastrointestinal
Gp	glycoprotein
GRF	gelatin–resorcinol–formaldehyde
GTN	glyceryl trinitrate
HIT	heparin-induced thrombocytopenia
IABP	intra-aortic balloon counterpulsation
IAC	interposed abdominal compression
IE	infective endocarditis
IHD	ischaemic heart disease
IMH	intramural haematoma
INR	international normalized ratio
IPG	impedance plethysmography
IRAD	International Registry of Acute Aortic Dissection
IV	intravenous
JVP	jugular venous pressure
LAD	left anterior descending (artery)
LIMA	left internal mammary artery
LMWH	low molecular weight heparin
LSD	lysergic acid diethylamide
LVF	left ventricular failure
MACE	major adverse cardiac event
MEN	multiple endocrine neoplasia
MI	myocardial infarction
MIC	minimum inhibitory concentration
MRI	magnetic resonance imaging
NPCT	non-penetrating cardiac trauma
NSTEMI	non-ST elevation MI
PAU	penetrating atherosclerotic ulceration
PCI	percutaneous coronary intervention
PE	pulmonary embolism
PEA	pulseless electrical activity
PLS	posterior leucoencephalopathy syndrome
PTCA	percutaneous transluminal coronary angioplasty
PTD	percutaneous thrombolytic device

PTFE	polytetrafluoroethylene
SLE	systemic lupus erythematosus
SVT	supraventricular tachycardia
TCA	tricyclic antidepressant
TIA	transient ischaemic attack
TOE	transoesophageal echocardiogram (echocardiography)
tPA	tissue plasminogen activator
TVR	target vessel revascularization
UFH	unfractionated heparin
V/Q	ventilation/perfusion
VF	ventricular fibrillation
VT	ventricular tachycardia
WCC	white cell count
WPW	Wolff–Parkinson–White (syndrome)

Myocardial infarction

1

Epidemiology

Myocardial infarction (MI) is a major cause of morbidity and mortality, affecting around 30 000 people per annum in the UK. In the last 30 years, mortality from MI has fallen by around a third in those aged less than 65 years of age. This reduction in mortality in younger individuals is due to a fall in the incidence of MI (reflecting improvements in nutrition, lifestyle and risk factor management) combined with an improved survival rate (reflecting improvements in medical therapy). This improvement in event rates and survival in younger individuals is offset by demographic changes in the population. Since MI is common and has a high mortality in older individuals and the population is rapidly ageing, the overall prevalence of MI related morbidity and mortality remains high.

Approximately 50 per cent of patients with MI die, with around two-thirds of the deaths occurring shortly after the onset of symptoms and before admission to hospital. Prior to the development of modern management strategies, hospital mortality after admission with MI was 30–40 per cent. After the introduction of coronary care units in the 1960s, outcome was improved, predominantly reflecting better treatment of arrhythmias. Current therapy has improved outcome further for younger patients who present early in the course of their MI, with hospital mortality rates of 5–10 per cent reported in the selected populations enrolled in large intervention trials. In routine clinical practice these very favourable mortality rates cannot be achieved (because of the increasing age of the population and contraindications to treatment in many patients) and hospital mortality in unselected UK populations remains around 15–20 per cent. Most patients who die before discharge do so in the first 48 hours after admission, usually due to cardiogenic shock consequent upon extensive left ventricular damage. Most patients who survive to hospital discharge do well, with 90 per cent surviving at least 1 year. Surviving patients who are at increased risk of early death can be identified by a series of adverse clinical and investigational features, and their prognosis improved by intervention.

Pathophysiology

Almost all episodes of MI are caused by thrombotic occlusion of a coronary artery occurring at the site of an unstable atherosclerotic lesion. Atherosclerosis is a disease of large and medium sized arteries, affecting predominantly the arterial intima. The precise mechanism responsible for the generation of atherosclerotic arterial disease remains open to debate, but it is clear that the extent and stability of atherosclerotic lesions is influenced by the common risk factors of smoking, hypertension, hyperlipidaemia and diabetes. There are a large number of other modifiable risk factors, such as homocysteine, antioxidants, fibrinogen, and psychosocial factors, which may play an important role in atherogenesis in some individuals. Individual susceptibility to the adverse effects of risk factors may relate to genetic predisposition or fetal adaptations that occur in response to the intrauterine environment. Fetal undernutrition leading to low birth weight and size is associated with the development of an adverse risk profile and a subsequent increase in the rate of MI. These findings suggest that adaptations made by the fetus in response to undernutrition leads to lifelong metabolic or structural changes that predispose to atherosclerosis.

Atherosclerotic plaques are complex structures consisting of a fibrous cap and a core of lipid, connective tissue and inflammatory cells. The morphology of plaques is variable, and those with a thin fibrous cap, a large lipid core and an increase in inflammatory activity are highly unstable. An increase in inflammatory activity within plaques may be triggered by systemic infections (such as *Chlamydia*, cytomegalovirus (CMV), *Helicobacter* or chronic dental sepsis) or stimuli such as stress, severe exercise and temperature change. Myocardial infarction is initiated when the fibrous cap of an unstable atherosclerotic lesion ruptures (in 75 per cent of cases) or the overlying endothelium erodes (in 25 per cent of cases). Plaque erosion is more common in females. Both mechanisms expose highly thrombogenic subendothelial and core components of the unstable plaque to the blood, leading to localized platelet adhesion, activation of the clotting mechanism, and formation of an intraluminal thrombus that occludes the coronary artery.

Most individuals with atherosclerotic coronary artery disease have a large number of minor lesions that do not significantly narrow the coronary lumen, as well as a smaller number of severe lesions. The severe lesions are more likely to intermittently limit antegrade blood flow during exercise (leading to stable angina). Thrombotic occlusion leading to MI is more likely to occur due to instability in one of the more numerous minor lesions (two-thirds of MIs are related to angiographically minor lesions). Acute MI associated with ST elevation usually occurs when total coronary occlusion develops rapidly and persists for at least 6–8 hours. Following coronary occlusion, myocardial cell necrosis develops after as little as 15 minutes. Cell necrosis continues for a variable time period (depending on the presence of collateral blood flow into the infarct zone, the reperfusion status of the infarct-related artery and the tolerance of the myocytes to ischaemia) but is largely complete after 6 hours of persistent coronary occlusion. Infarcts can be classified as small (<10 per cent of the left ventricle), medium (10–30 per cent of the left ventricle) or large (>30 per cent of the left ventricle). Short-lived or partial occlusions are usually associated with ST depression or T-wave changes, and present as unstable angina or non-ST segment elevation MI. When plaque disruption is limited, vessel occlusion is predominantly due to thrombotic occlusion, and thrombolytic therapy usually restores antegrade blood flow, limiting infarct size and improving outcome. In some individuals, plaque disruption is extensive, and luminal occlusion predominantly due to mechanical obstruction by the components of the disrupted plaque. In these patients, thrombolysis may not resolve the mechanical lumen obstruction, leading to failure to reperfuse and a poor clinical outcome. These lesions are more easily treated by coronary angioplasty.

A number of factors that can trigger the onset of MI have been identified, acting by initiating plaque rupture or promoting thrombus formation. Some patients report heavy physical exertion or mental stress shortly before the onset of MI. Circadian variation in coagulation and autonomic nervous system activity contribute to an increased incidence of MI in the morning. Irrespective of this, the risk of an individual episode of exercise or stress precipitating the onset of MI is low, and most episodes have no identifiable direct triggers.

Diagnosis

Background

Acute MI with chest pain is a common reason for patients attending hospital. Around 50 per cent of patients presenting with chest pain have an acute coronary syndrome (evolving MI or unstable angina) as the cause of their symptoms, requiring hospitalization and intensive medical therapy. The other 50 per cent of patients have other cardiac and non-cardiac causes for their symptoms, and require a different management approach. This section gives guidelines on diagnosing acute MI, and differentiating it from other common causes of chest pain.

The diagnosis of evolving acute MI is usually made using a combination of clinical and electrocardiographic features. Cardiac enzyme studies are then used to confirm or refute the diagnosis, and to quantify the magnitude of myocardial necrosis that has occurred. As a general principle, all patients with symptoms that may be due to an evolving MI should be admitted to hospital. These patients should preferably be admitted to CCU, as they are at high risk of early adverse events and benefit from intensive therapy.

Clinical features

The pain associated with evolving MI is typically retrosternal, crushing and severe. Pain often radiates to the neck, arms or back. There is often associated nausea, sweating and vomiting related to the release of toxins from injured myocardial cells and autonomic activation. The pain associated with MI usually lasts at least 20 minutes and is not usually affected by changes in posture, movement or respiration. The pain can be atypical (sited in the epigastrium, neck, arms or back or unusual in character). Particularly with inferior infarction, the pain can be difficult to distinguish from dyspepsia. In some patients, the pain is minimal or absent, with the dominant symptoms consisting of nausea, vomiting, dyspnoea, weakness, dizziness, or syncope (or a combination of these). In some patients, MI occurs without any symptoms, when it is recognized coincidentally (and often retrospectively) by the presence of abnormalities on the ECG or other imaging modalities.

Electrocardiographic changes

The majority of patients with evolving MI will have an abnormal ECG at some stage. An initial normal ECG does not rule out the diagnosis, as ECG changes can develop, evolve and resolve rapidly. Patients with a suggestive history and a normal ECG should be admitted and the ECG monitored at regular intervals; if ECG changes then develop, appropriate treatment can be initiated. The most common ECG abnormality (present at some stage in around 70 per cent of patients with chest pain and evolving MI) is ST elevation. In patients with this type of evolving MI:

- ST elevation develops rapidly (30–60 seconds) after coronary occlusion, and is usually associated with prolonged total occlusion of a coronary artery.
- The ST elevation resolves over several hours in response to spontaneous or therapeutic coronary reperfusion. Persistent ST elevation is a sign of failure to reperfuse, and is associated with a large infarct and an adverse prognosis. T-wave inversion, pathological Q waves and loss of R waves often develop in the infarct zone when reperfusion has been late or incomplete, indicating the presence of extensive myocardial necrosis. When successful reperfusion occurs early in the course of an evolving ST elevation MI, there may be little myocardial necrosis, preservation of the R waves and no Q-wave formation.

In a small proportion of patients with chest pain and evolving MI (around 5 per cent) the presenting ECG demonstrates bundle branch block (usually left). This is commonly associated with extensive anterior infarction and a poor prognosis.

In a substantial number of patients with chest pain and evolving MI (around 25 per cent) the initial ECG shows ST depression, T-wave changes, or other non-specific abnormalities. In younger patients, this pattern of non-ST elevation MI is often associated with limited necrosis and localized coronary artery disease. Older patients with widespread severe ST depression often have multivessel disease and a poor prognosis.

The distribution of ECG changes provides some information on the area of myocardium involved:

- Changes in V2–V6 indicate anterior ischaemia or necrosis in the territory of the left anterior descending (LAD) artery. Extensive infarction in this territory is associated with a high risk of heart failure, arrhythmias, mechanical complications and early death (Figure 1.1).
- Changes in I, aVL, V5 and V6 indicate lateral ischaemia or necrosis in the territory of the circumflex artery or diagonal branches of the LAD (Figure 1.2). Infarction in this territory has a better prognosis than extensive anterior infarction.
- Changes in II, III and aVF indicate inferior ischaemia or necrosis in the territory of the right coronary artery (Figure 1.3). Compared with patients with extensive anterior infarction, these patients have a lower incidence of heart failure, an increased incidence of bradyarrhythmias (since AV nodal ischaemia or vagal activation often accompanies occlusion of the right coronary artery) and a relatively good prognosis.
- Tall R waves in V1–V3 associated with ST depression indicate ischaemia or necrosis in the posterior wall, often associated with circumflex or right coronary artery occlusion (Figure 1.4).

A large infarct is indicated by the presence of extensive ST change occurring in multiple ECG leads.

Diagnostic biochemical markers

Cardiac enzyme studies are employed to substantiate or refute a provisional diagnosis of MI, and guide further therapy. Myocardial necrosis results in the release of intracellular proteins, which can be detected in blood samples. Measurement of total creatine kinase (CK) level has been employed as a common biochemical test in patients with suspected MI, with a temporally related increase to more than twice the upper limit of normal regarded as diagnostic. Creatine kinase is widely distributed in non-cardiac tissues, and therefore has a significant rate of false-positive results. Troponin T and I are intracellular proteins

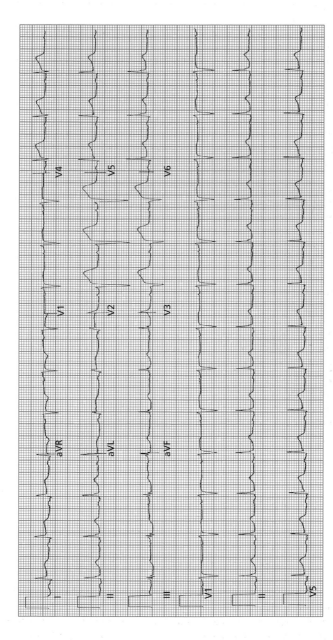

Figure 1.1 Anterolateral myocardial infarction. Note ST elevation in leads V2–V5, I and aVL.

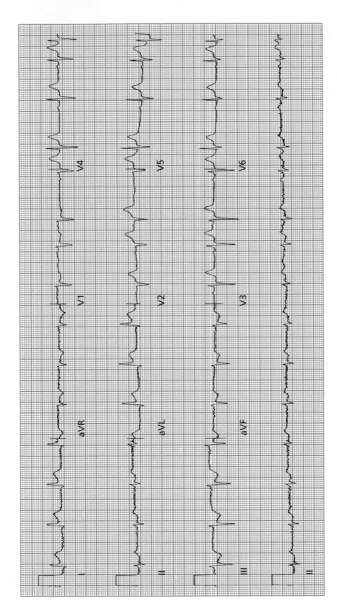

Figure 1.2 High lateral myocardial infarction. Note the ST elevation in leads 1 and aVL with reciprocal changes in the inferior leads. Coronary angiography demonstrated a 95 per cent stenosis in a high diagonal branch.

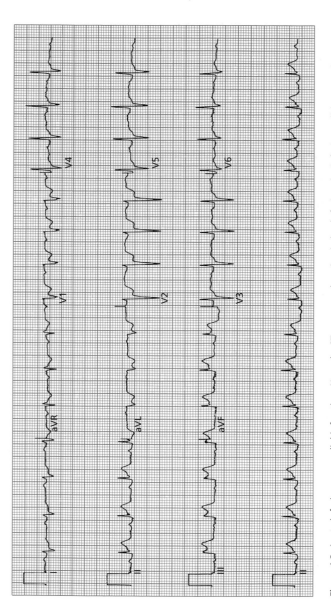

Figure 1.3 Acute inferior myocardial infarction. Note the ST segment elevation in leads facing the inferior wall (II, III, aVF). Reciprocal changes are seen in diametrically opposed leads (I and aVL) located in the same (frontal) plane.

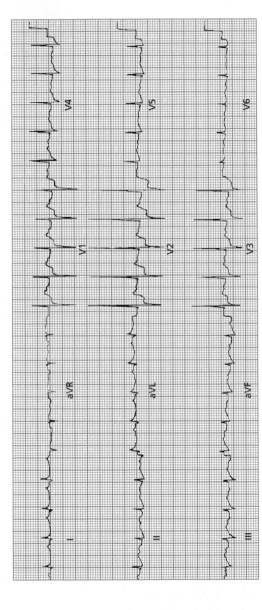

Figure 1.4 Posterior wall myocardial infarction. Note the tall R waves in leads V1–V3 associated with ST depression.

involved in the regulation of the cellular contractile process. Specific cardiac isoforms of these troponins can be detected and measured, and the presence of these biomarkers is therefore a specific indication that myocardial necrosis has occurred. As well as their specificity, cardiac troponins are highly sensitive, with detectable elevations occurring after necrosis of less than 1 g myocardial tissue. Troponins are detectable 3–4 hours after the onset of infarction, peak around 36–48 hours, and can remain elevated for up to 2 weeks. False-positive results are rare, but can be due to:

- renal failure
- myocarditis
- pulmonary embolism
- acute heart failure
- cardiac trauma
- septicaemia
- cardiotoxic drugs
- tachycardia with haemodynamic compromise.

Because of their sensitivity and specificity, troponins are now the recommended serum marker for detecting myocardial necrosis. Any patient who demonstrates a typical rise and gradual fall of troponin in association with ischaemic symptoms or ECG changes should be diagnosed as having had a definite MI.

Other causes of chest pain

Unstable angina is as common as acute MI, and has a similar pathophysiology and prognosis. In patients who present with intermittent chest pain and ST depression or T-wave changes, the final diagnosis can only be clarified when the results of a cardiac enzyme series are available. Patients with unstable angina have symptoms of ischaemic cardiac pain that:

- occurs at rest or on minimal exertion;
- is unresponsive or poorly responsive to nitrate administration;
- occurs with increasing frequency, and may be severe and/or prolonged.

The ECG may be normal or demonstrate variable degrees of ST depression or T-wave inversion. The management of patients with unstable angina is dealt with in detail in Chapter 2.

Non-cardiac chest pain can arise from:

- the aorta in acute dissection. The pain of aortic dissection is severe and of sudden onset; it is tearing in nature, often radiates to the back, and may be associated with hypertension, aortic regurgitation, neurological signs and pulse deficits.

- the pleura in pneumonia, pulmonary embolism or pneumothorax. Pain arising from the pleura is unilateral, sharp and stabbing, and worse on inspiration. There may be associated signs of pneumonia, pulmonary embolus or deep venous thrombosis. The majority of patients with pulmonary embolus have no ECG changes apart from a tachycardia or atrial fibrillation. ECG changes of $S_1Q_3T_3$ or right heart strain are associated with large emboli and are often transient and easily missed. In spontaneous pneumothorax, there may be central chest pain with few auscultatory signs. Spontaneous pneumothorax is a strong possibility in patients with chronic obstructive pulmonary disease (COPD) who present with chest pain and dyspnoea in the absence of ECG evidence of acute myocardial ischaemia. A chest x-ray is vital to rule out the presence of air in the pleural space.
- the upper gastrointestinal (GI) tract in oesophageal reflux, peptic ulcer disease or cholelithiasis. Dyspeptic pain arising from the upper GI tract is usually burning in nature, may have a clear relationship to posture or food, and is often relieved by antacids. Oesophageal pain may, however, be very similar to the pain of cardiac ischaemia. Exercise-induced oesophageal pain mimicking angina has been well described. In some individuals, oesophageal spasm may occur in association with ST segment change. Nitrates and calcium antagonists will relieve the pain of oesophageal spasm. Correct diagnosis in these difficult patients requires coronary arteriography, investigations to rule out coronary spasm, myocardial perfusion imaging and ambulatory oesophageal pH and pressure monitoring.
- the pericardium in pericarditis. Pericardial pain is retrosternal, sharp, eased by sitting forward, and may worsen with inspiration. It is commonly seen following MI, or in a young adult with acute post-viral pericarditis. A pericardial rub is common, although it may be intermittent. Diagnostic widespread concave ST elevation may be present.
- the bones and muscles in musculoskeletal disorders. Musculoskeletal chest pain is usually unilateral, localized and sharp. It is exacerbated by movement or local pressure. There may be a history of trauma.
- the skin in acute dermatological conditions. Acute skin conditions can (rarely) produce chest pain. The unilateral pain of shingles precedes the rash, and may confuse the unwary.
- outside the chest cavity. For example, referred pain from the neck. Pain referred from the cervical or thoracic spine will have features of musculoskeletal chest pain.

Since acute chest pain can have many possible causes, a careful history and comprehensive physical examination along with inspection of the ECG and chest x-ray are mandatory in all cases, where diagnostic uncertainty exists.

Risk assessment in patients with acute chest pain

Patients who present with chest pain and ischaemic ECG changes require admission and appropriate treatment. Even if the ECG is normal, a good history of an unstable pattern of ischaemic chest pain (particularly if rest pain lasting for more than 15 minutes occurs) indicates that admission is required for further evaluation and treatment; these patients have an unstable coronary syndrome until proven otherwise. A firm alternative diagnosis will be obvious (for example, pneumothorax with an abnormal chest x-ray, or pericarditis with widespread concave ST elevation) in some patients.

In a proportion of patients, however, the history will be non-specific, clinical examination unremarkable, the ECG will be normal or nondiagnostic and it will be impossible to rule out an acute coronary syndrome on clinical grounds alone. In these patients, measurement of cardiac specific troponins is of value. Troponin levels should be measured on arrival and after a further 12 hours. Around 10–20 per cent of these patients will have detectable troponin elevation, indicating that their pain is cardiac in origin. These patients have an acute coronary syndrome, are at increased risk of an early adverse cardiac event, and require hospital admission and appropriate treatment. If two appropriately timed troponin tests are negative, the risk of an adverse cardiac event occurring early is low, and the patient can be safely discharged to be further investigated as an out-patient.

Initial treatment

Background

Patients with evolving MI often do not request medical aid until symptoms have been present for more than 1 hour. This patient delay occurs at the most critical time in the course of the illness, when pain is often severe and the risk of ventricular tachyarrhythmias and cardiac arrest is high. Although mass public education campaigns may shorten the duration of this patient delay, they have had no significant impact on outcome. Once a patient with suspected acute MI arrives in hospital, rapid processing is necessary to establish an early diagnosis and allow effective emergency care to be instituted. Patients who present to the emergency department with possible acute MI should be reviewed as soon as possible by an appropriately trained doctor. The initial assessment should be rapid, and aimed at establishing the diagnosis, assessing the haemodynamic state and determining suitability for reperfusion therapy. Comprehensive history taking and examination can be deferred until the patient has received appropriate emergency care and is stable on the Coronary Care Unit (CCU). Patients with clear-cut clinical features of acute MI and an ECG that demonstrates ST elevation or bundle branch block should enter a 'fast track' system, designed to ensure that they receive appropriate emergency care and that reperfusion therapy is instituted within 90 minutes of the initial call for medical assistance. A successful fast track system is only possible if medical staff respond rapidly to calls from the emergency department, and the aim should be to review patients with a suggestive history and ECG changes within 10 minutes of their arrival. The 'door-to-needle' time should not exceed 20 minutes for fast track patients.

Emergency care

In a patient with chest pain lasting for more than 15 minutes that is not responding to sublingual nitrates and with electrocardiographic ST elevation or left bundle branch block, a provisional diagnosis of acute MI can confidently be reached and emergency therapy initiated. If the clinical features are atypical and the ECG is equivocal but there is a strong suspicion of evolving myocardial infarction, treatment with heparin, beta-blockers, nitrates and aspirin should be instituted. Thrombolytic therapy should not be given to patients with a normal ECG, T-wave inversion or ST depression; there is no evidence that lytic therapy will be of benefit in these cases. The patient should be admitted to the CCU, and repeated ECG recordings or, if available, continuous ST segment monitoring performed. If ST segment elevation or bundle branch block develops, thrombolytic therapy should be administered.

Having reached a provisional diagnosis of acute MI, emergency care consists of relief of pain, breathlessness and anxiety, and administration of reperfusion therapy and aspirin as early as possible. The priorities are to:

- establish venous access with a large-bore cannula in an arm vein providing ready access for drug administration, and institute rhythm monitoring to aid in the rapid detection and treatment of arrhythmias.

- provide adequate analgesia, which is vital. Uncontrolled pain and anxiety are associated with sympathetic activation, with resultant detrimental effects on cardiac performance, oxygen consumption and the arrhythmia threshold. Intravenous opioids are indicated to provide rapid relief of pain. Intramuscular injections should be avoided, as they have a slower onset of action, are associated with unpredictable absorption, may cause a haematoma if thrombolytic therapy is given, and can affect CK estimations. The agent of choice is diamorphine 2.5–5.0 mg by slow intravenous (IV) injection, with metoclopramide 10 mg IV as an anti-emetic. The dose should be repeated every 5 minutes until adequate analgesia is achieved. If repeated administration of diamorphine fails to relieve the pain, intravenous beta-blockers or nitrates should be considered. Respiratory depression produced by diamorphine can, if necessary, be rapidly reversed by naloxone.
- treat pulmonary oedema with IV frusemide 40–80 mg. If pulmonary oedema is severe, an IV nitrate infusion (as detailed in Appendix A) should be commenced.
- consider supplemental oxygen. Hypoxia is common in patients with evolving infarction, and may increase myocardial necrosis or have adverse metabolic effects. Supplemental oxygen will optimize oxygen delivery and limit ischaemia, and should be given to all patients with breathlessness or features of heart failure. Since hypoxia may be present in 20 per cent of patients with an initially uncomplicated infarct, pulse oximetry should be instituted in all cases, and oxygen given if saturation falls below 93 per cent. High concentration (up to 60 per cent) oxygen can be given via an MC mask if necessary. If the patient has COPD, therapy with 24 or 28 per cent oxygen via a venti-mask is commenced, and the concentration adjusted depending on blood gas measurements to prevent CO_2 retention in patients who are reliant on hypoxic drive to maintain ventilation.
- commence treatment with aspirin (in an initial dose of at least 160 mg) in the emergency department. Aspirin should be given prior to reperfusion therapy, as it may aid clot lysis and improve efficacy if thrombolysis is employed.
- institute reperfusion therapy. In most UK patients this will consist of thrombolysis. It is important to commence thrombolytic therapy as early as possible. Mortality in patients treated within an hour of the onset of symptoms is only 1.2 per cent, compared with 8.7 per cent for those treated later.

Having established intravenous access and continuous rhythm monitoring and administered analgesia, oxygen, aspirin and thrombolytic therapy, the patient can be transferred to the CCU for further evaluation and therapy.

Early investigation and treatment on the CCU

Following transfer to the CCU, a full history and examination can be performed. The indications for intravenous beta-blockers and urgent percutaneous transluminal coronary angioplasty (PTCA) should be reviewed. Electrolytes, glucose, blood count and chest x-ray are urgently obtained. Blood is sent for routine estimation of cardiac enzymes and cholesterol. A variety of therapeutic options have recently been evaluated. This section discusses their relative merits and indications for use.

Hypokalaemia

Hypokalaemia is common in patients with acute infarction, and is related to prior treatment with diuretics or catecholamine effects on electrolyte handling. Hypokalaemia is associated with myocardial electrical instability [the incidence of ventricular fibrillation (VF) may be as high as 15 per cent in infarcts associated with a potassium of 3.0–3.5 mmol/L, and 5 per cent or less in infarcts associated with a potassium of 4.5–5.0 mmol/L] and should be corrected. If serum potassium is below 4.0 mmol/L in the absence of an important arrhythmia, then oral potassium supplements are given (e.g. SLOW K, three tablets three times daily, providing approximately 120 mmol potassium daily) and potassium re-checked after 12–18 hours. If ventricular arrhythmias occur in association with a serum potassium of less than 4.0 mmol/L, intravenous potassium is given as detailed in Appendix A, re-checking serum levels after 3 hours to ensure that potassium levels have risen to greater than 4.0 mmol/L.

Magnesium therapy

A number of small studies (including LIMIT-2) suggested that routine administration of magnesium may reduce mortality following acute infarction by beneficial effects on heart rate, contractility, electrical stability and platelet activity. The routine use of magnesium was therefore examined in almost 60 000 patients in the ISIS-4 study, and this showed that treatment had no beneficial effect on mortality. Subgroup analysis showed no benefit even when magnesium was given early, or to patients who did not receive thrombolytic therapy. These results were confirmed in the recent MAGIC trial of over 6000 patients. There is therefore no good evidence to support the routine use of magnesium in patients with evolving acute MI. Magnesium is, however, still indicated for the treatment of arrhythmias.

Nitrate therapy

Nitrates have a number of potentially beneficial effects (systemic vaso-dilatation and coronary artery dilatation), and small early studies suggested that their routine administration to patients with acute infarction may reduce mortality. The ISIS-4 and GISSI-3 trials investigated routine nitrate use in a total of almost 80 000 patients, and found no substantial beneficial effect on mortality. Although nitrates are safe and effective in the treatment of post-infarction ischaemia or heart failure, they should not routinely be administered to uncomplicated patients.

Hyperglycaemia

Patients with pre-existing diabetes have an increased risk of ischaemic heart disease, and an unfavourable prognosis following acute MI. Patients who have no history of diabetes but an elevated glucose on admission also have a poor prognosis. The high mortality may be related to the occurrence of autonomic neuropathy, pre-existing ventricular dysfunction or due to detrimental myocardial cellular changes induced by diabetes. Additionally, sympathetic activation will induce insulin resistance and hyperglycaemia in susceptible patients, increasing the release of non-esterified fatty acids, which augment myocardial oxygen consumption, depress contractility and increase the risk of heart failure. A strategy of controlling elevated plasma glucose by insulin infusion followed by subcutaneous injections in hyperglycaemic patients with acute MI could prevent these adverse metabolic effects, and was investigated in over 600 patients randomized in the DIGAMI trial. Treatment with intravenous insulin reduced mortality by around 40 per cent. The maximum reduction in mortality occurred in patients who had not previously received insulin therapy, and were at low risk of death on the basis of clinical criteria. On the basis of these trial data, it is recommended that all patients with an admission glucose <11 mmol/L should be commenced on a sliding scale intravenous insulin infusion with the infusion rate adjusted to maintain blood glucose in the range 7–11 mmol/L, in combination with 500 mL of 5 per cent dextrose infused over 24 hours. Oral hypoglycaemic agents should be withdrawn. The infusion should be continued for at least 24 hours, or until the patient is clinically stable, and followed by at least 3 months of treatment with subcutaneous insulin.

Prophylactic antiarrhythmic therapy

Ventricular tachyarrhythmias are an important cause of death early after the onset of MI. Class I antiarrhythmic drugs can suppress these arrhythmias, but this beneficial effect may be offset by adverse effects such as the induction of bradyarrhythmias, induction of tachyarrhythmias and depression of ventricular function. A meta-analysis of more than 200 000 patients treated with prophylactic class I drugs showed no beneficial effects on mortality. On the basis of these trial data, routine prophylactic therapy with class I antiarrhythmic drugs early in the course of evolving MI is not recommended.

Pre-existing drug therapy

Patients admitted with evolving acute MI are often already on treatment with oral beta-blockers for pre-existing angina or hypertension. Given the beneficial effects of beta-blockers following infarction and the potential adverse effects associated with abrupt beta-blocker withdrawal, administration of these agents should continue uninterrupted unless important heart failure or a symptomatic bradyarrhythmia develops. Combined oral contraceptives are associated with an increased risk of thromboembolism and should be withdrawn.

Thrombolysis

Background

Thrombolytic therapy for acute MI was first used in 1958. Debate about its efficacy continued until 1986, when the publication of the first GISSI study clearly demonstrated the value of streptokinase. By the mid-1990s, more than 100 000 patients had been randomized into a series of large-scale thrombolytic trials, that have helped to optimize the use of thrombolytic drugs. These large-scale trials have demonstrated that:

- thrombolysis produces an important time-dependent reduction in mortality. Treatment within the first hour after symptom onset can prevent irreversible myocardial necrosis from progressing, and abort an evolving infarct. Treatment within the first 6 hours of symptom onset limits infarct size and reduces mortality by 25 per cent. Treatment between 6 and 12 hours may help to salvage some ischaemic myocardium (particularly in the border zone of the infarct) and reduces mortality by about 10 per cent. Although patients treated 12–24 hours after symptom onset may still benefit from opening an occluded artery (which may improve the healing process and limit ventricular dilatation), there is no evidence that mortality is reduced. Based on this first series of trials, thrombolytic therapy reduces 1-month mortality by 17 per cent, preventing 18 deaths for every 1000 patients treated. This mortality benefit is maintained in the long term, with 10-year survival rates substantially improved in treated patients. Newer, more efficacious agents have improved on these 1-month and 10-year survival figures.

- mortality reduction is present regardless of age, sex or infarct site.
- aspirin has an additive beneficial effect of similar magnitude to that produced by thrombolysis, and should be given to all patients with evolving MI.
- the concurrent use of heparin and thrombolytic therapy has been extensively studied. There are no beneficial effects apparent when intravenous or subcutaneous heparin is used with streptokinase or with early rt-PA (alteplase) regimens but the risk of bleeding complications is increased. For accelerated rt-PA and the newer plasminogen activators, heparin [controlled by regular activated partial thromboplastin time (aPTT) monitoring] reduces coronary re-occlusion rates, and should be given for 48 hours.
- thrombolysis increases the risk of stroke in the first 24 hours after treatment, but this is offset by the much larger reduction in cardiac deaths with treatment. Stroke risk is greater in older patients (over 75 years of age) and those with systolic hypertension. Bleeding from other sites can occur (particularly at the site of vascular punctures) and may require blood transfusion.
- the evidence for a beneficial effect in patients with ST elevation or bundle branch block is strong. There is no clear evidence that patients with ST depression, T-wave inversion or a normal ECG derive benefit. These patients are, however, at a similar risk of bleeding complications, and should not initially receive thrombolytic therapy. For these patients, frequent or continuous ECGs should be obtained, and thrombolysis only administered if ST elevation evolves.

On the basis of this large body of data from randomized trials, all patients who present within 12 hours of the onset of symptoms of an evolving MI, and have ST elevation or bundle branch block, should receive thrombolytic therapy if there are no contraindications. Because beneficial effects are time dependent, thrombolysis should be administered as early as possible. Patients who do not meet these strict criteria should not be treated (at least initially), thereby limiting the risk of side effects in patients with limited potential for benefit.

Selection of thrombolytic agents

The relative efficacy of different thrombolytic agents and regimens has been compared in several trials. The early studies showed similar efficacy for streptokinase and non-accelerated rt-PA regimens. In 1993, the Global Utilisation of STreptokinase for Occluded coronary arteries (GUSTO) trial reported. This trial compared four different streptokinase and rt-PA regimens, and demonstrated that an accelerated rt-PA regimen (given over 90 minutes rather than 3 hours) with subsequent aPTT-controlled intravenous heparin was superior, improving early coronary patency rates from around 30 per cent with streptokinase to 50 per cent with rt-PA and reducing death rates. Most of the beneficial effect on mortality was obtained in patients with anterior infarction treated within 6 hours of symptom onset.

The thrombolytic regimens used in early studies have a number of disadvantages. Streptokinase has only limited efficacy (and may be totally ineffective in the presence of pre-existing antibodies) and accelerated rt-PA has a complex dosing regimen. These problems have led to the development of three new plasminogen activators, produced by bioengineering techniques applied to rt-PA. These three compounds, reteplase (r-PA), tenecteplase (TNK) and lanoteplase (n-PA) have a longer half life than the original compound, and can therefore be administered in single or double bolus regimens, simplifying clinical usage. The simple administration regimens of these new plasminogen activators has been shown to shorten door-to-needle times in observational trials, compared with the more complex dosing regimens of other agents. The relative efficacy of these new agents has been compared to older thrombolytic agents in a series of trials enrolling more than 50 000 patients (INJECT, INTIME-2, GUSTO-3, ASSENT-2). These trials show that TNK has equivalent efficacy to rt-PA, whilst reteplase has at least equivalent efficacy to streptokinase. The lanoteplase regimen used in the INTIME-2 trial was associated with a substantial increase in intracerebral bleeding, and this agent is not currently available for use in the UK.

The combination of thrombolysis and more potent platelet inhibition (with intravenous IIb/IIIa receptor blockers) or antithrombotic therapy (with low molecular weight heparin) has been studied. Despite the promising results of small early trials suggesting that these regimens improve early patency rates, effects on mortality have been disappointing. In more than 20 000 patients enrolled in GUSTO-5 and ASSENT-3, there was no reduction in mortality for patients treated with combination therapy, although early recurrent ischaemia was reduced. In both trials there was an increase in bleeding complications, particularly in the elderly. In ASSENT-3, low molecular weight heparin had a similar effect as IIb/IIIa inhibition for the prevention of early recurrent ischaemia, with a less pronounced effect on the rate of major bleeding.

On the basis of this series of trials, accelerated rt-PA or TNK with concomitant heparin are the regimens with the best record for mortality reduction. Plasminogen activators are preferred in patients who have a low blood pressure at presentation (because of the risk of a further fall in blood pressure induced by streptokinase), and in patients who have previously received streptokinase (since the induction of neutralizing antibodies may limit the efficacy of a second dose). The modified plasminogen activators have the simplest dosing regimens, helping to reduce door-to-needle time. The choice of thrombolytic agent is dictated by several factors (efficacy, administration regimen, cost), and the administration regimens for all agents currently licensed for use in the UK are provided in Appendix A. Intravenous IIb/IIIa receptor blockers and low molecular weight heparins used in conjunction with thrombolysis have favourable effects on early recurrent ischaemia, but no proven mortality benefit. Low molecular weight heparin has the advantage of ease of administration and may become standard therapy if further studies confirm the results of ASSENT-3.

Inclusion criteria

Patients suitable for thrombolysis are selected on the basis of the following criteria. The chosen thrombolytic agent should be administered without delay, and aspirin should be given prior to thrombolysis in all cases.

- Presentation within 12 hours of onset of ischaemic cardiac pain in a patient with:
  - ST segment elevation of at least 2 mm in two adjacent chest leads;
  - ST segment elevation of 1 mm in two adjacent limb leads;
  - true posterior infarction or new bundle branch block.
- Presentation 12–24 hours after onset of pain in the presence of ongoing symptoms and ECG evidence of evolving infarction.

Exclusion criteria

These continue to evolve, and are in general decreasing as our experience with thrombolytic agents increases. At present there are few absolute contraindications. Many are now regarded as relative, to be interpreted within the clinical context. Criteria include:

- known coagulation disorder, including uncontrolled anticoagulation therapy;
- active peptic ulceration, varices or recent GI haemorrhage (dyspepsia alone is not a contraindication);
- severe hypertension (systolic >180 mmHg and/or diastolic <110 mmHg);
- traumatic cardiopulmonary resuscitation (CPR) (CPR performed by trained staff is not regarded as a contraindication);
- recent internal bleeding from any site (menstruation is not an absolute contraindication);
- previous haemorrhagic stroke at any time;
- ischaemic stroke within the last year;
- transient ischaemic attack (TIA) in last 3 months;
- surgery, major trauma or head injury within the last month;
- pregnancy;
- diabetic retinopathy (now only a relative contraindication, as the risk of intraocular bleeding is very small and the potential benefit of thrombolysis in diabetics far outweighs this risk).

If in doubt about administering thrombolysis, a senior colleague should be consulted. If bleeding risk outweighs perceived benefits, primary PTCA is a safer and highly effective alternative.

Complications

ALLERGY

Allergic reactions to streptokinase are due to the effect of pre-existing anti-streptococcal antibodies. Mild urticarial reactions are the most common allergic response, and should be treated with 200 mg IV hydrocortisone and 10 mg IV chlorpheniramine. If a more severe reaction with bronchospasm occurs, 250–500 µg of intramuscular adrenaline should be administered along with nebulized bronchodilators. Major anaphylaxis is very rare (0.1 per cent). If this occurs, with associated cardiovascular collapse, 5 mL of 1:10 000 adrenaline IV is first-line therapy, followed by rapid volume loading with IV plasma expanders, steroids and antihistamines. Allergic reactions to the newer plasminogen activators are very rare.

HAEMORRHAGE

Minor bleeding at venepuncture sites is relatively common, but rarely requires any specific therapy other than direct compression at the site. Major haemorrhagic episodes requiring transfusion are rare. If a major bleed occurs consider the following action:

- stop thrombolytic infusion (or heparin);
- reverse heparin with protamine sulphate (10 mg per 1000 u heparin);
- give two units of fresh frozen plasma immediately;
- consider the administration of tranexamic acid 10 mg/kg by slow IV injection.

HYPOTENSION

Hypotensive reactions to thrombolytic infusion can occur with any agent, but are more common with streptokinase. They should be treated initially by tilting the patient's head down and, in the case of strepto-kinase, the infusion should be slowed down or, if necessary, halted for 5 minutes. It can usually be successfully restarted when the blood pres-sure recovers. Atropine 0.6 mg IV can be given if a bradycardia is also present. If the hypotension persists and is clearly associated with the infusion, then the drug should be stopped, and a plasminogen activator substituted for streptokinase, as it is less likely to cause hypotension. In the case of severe persistent hypotension, fluids and inotropes can be administered cautiously if necessary.

CEREBROVASCULAR EVENTS

The overall incidence of stroke is only minimally increased, since throm-bolytic therapy causes a slight increase in cerebral haemorrhages, which is offset by a reduction in cerebral infarcts. Plasminogen activators are associated with a greater risk of haemorrhagic stroke than streptokinase. Stroke is more common in older patients. If a stroke occurs, thrombolytic or anticoagulant therapy should be discontinued. A computed tomo-graphy (CT) scan and neurological opinion will help to determine the mechanism of the stroke and guide therapy.

Failed reperfusion

Detection and implications of failed reperfusion

Patients treated with thrombolysis who achieve effective reperfusion have a good prognosis, with hospital mortality rates of less than 5 per cent.

Achievement of successful reperfusion is associated with infarct artery patency, restoration of rapid antegrade blood flow into a patent micro-circulation and resolution of chest pain. In a substantial proportion of patients, reperfusion fails. In some of these patients the infarct-related artery is persistently occluded by an extensively disrupted plaque or residual thrombus. In other patients (particularly those treated late) platelet microthrombi or capillary disruption prevent reperfusion of myocardium at the tissue level despite restoration of blood flow in the epicardial infarct-related artery. Failure of reperfusion is associated with continuing chest pain, extensive infarction, electrical and haemody-namic instability, mechanical complications and a poor prognosis.

Detecting failed reperfusion in current clinical practice is based on serial evaluation of ST segments. Persistence of ST elevation occurs in about one-third of patients, and is associated with failure of reperfusion due to one of the above mechanisms. Patients with persistent ST eleva-tion have a poor prognosis. In the 1398 patients enrolled in the INJECT trial, those with no ST resolution had a 17.5 per cent hospital mortality, those with partial resolution a 4.3 per cent mortality and those with total resolution a 2.5 per cent mortality. On the basis of these data, all patients should have an ECG recorded 90–180 minutes after commencing throm-bolysis. Patients who have less than 50 per cent ST segment resolution in the infarct zone should be considered for further therapy.

Management of failed reperfusion

The evidence available to guide optimal management of failed reper-fusion is limited. Until further evidence from large-scale clinical trials is available, the strategy chosen will depend on local resources and pref-erences. The options are:

- Monitor the patient closely and use optimal adjunctive therapy (such as beta-blockers and heart failure therapy).
- Administer repeat thrombolysis. There is some evidence that this reduces infarct size, but the risk of intracranial haemorrhage is doubled. Repeat thrombolysis may only be effective if measurement of fibrinogen levels indicates that initial treatment has failed to achieve a systemic lytic state (with raised fibrinogen levels, particularly following streptokinase administration, indicating that a systemic lytic state has not been achieved).
- Perform rescue PTCA. The limited data available to date (involving around 700 patients) suggest that rescue PTCA may reduce infarct size and improve outcome.

Decision-making is difficult in this complex area. Therapy needs to be tailored to each individual patient, taking into account age (which influences stroke risk) size of infarct, co-morbidity, time since onset of symptoms (which influence the amount of viable myocardium that can possibly be salvaged) and local facilities. For haemodynamically stable patients with a small infarct (ST elevation in a maximum of three leads), particularly if they present more than 6 hours after the symptom onset, the risks of rescue PTCA or repeat thrombolysis probably outweigh the benefits, and a conservative approach is a reasonable option. For patients with failure to reperfuse who present early (within 6 hours) in the course of a large infarct (marked ST elevation in multiple leads), particularly if accompanied by haemodynamic compromise, repeated thrombolysis or rescue PTCA is more justified.

Recurrent ischaemia

Following successful thrombolytic therapy, patients are often left with a residual high grade stenosis. The strategy of performing angiography followed by revascularization as a routine in all patients has been evaluated in 4000 patients randomized in a series of trials (TAMI-I, ECSG, TIMI-2A, TIMI-2B and SWIFT). Early non-selective intervention was not associated with beneficial effects on left ventricular function, recurrent ischaemia or mortality. On the basis of these data, asymptomatic post-MI patients who have a satisfactory risk factor profile should be managed conservatively.

In up to one-third of post-infarct patients, recurrent ischaemia occurs after thrombolysis, and is associated with increased hospital mortality. In most instances, early recurrent ischaemia is related to further thrombus formation at the site of the original unstable atherosclerotic plaque. There are limited trial data available to guide treatment in these patients.

For patients who have early re-infarction with chest pain and further ST elevation, the options are:

- immediate cardiac catheterization followed by PTCA if possible. Intra-aortic balloon pumping may help to reduce the procedure-related morbidity.
- repeat thrombolysis.

The preferred option will depend on local facilities, expertise, patient age and co-morbidity. For patients with recurrent infarction and haemodynamic instability, coronary angiography and PTCA offers the best chance of improving prognosis. Hospital mortality rate after re infarction is in the range of 40 per cent.

For patients who have a pattern of post-infarction unstable angina with recurrent chest pain in association with dynamic ST segment depression or T wave changes:

- Treat with heparin. If the patient is already on intravenous heparin, ensure anticoagulation is in the therapeutic range by checking aPTT.
- Optimize anti-ischaemic therapy with intravenous nitrates and beta-blockers.

Patients with post-infarction unstable angina require cardiac catheterization and revascularization. Cardiac catheterization should be performed in all patients who are suitable for a revascularization procedure. Revascularization by PTCA is the preferred option if technically suitable culprit lesions are present. Many of these patients, however, have extensive, severe proximal multi-vessel or left main stem disease, and may require a coronary artery bypass graft (CABG). The mortality rate of CABG performed early after MI is increased in a time-dependent fashion; if the patient can be stabilized with intensive medical therapy and surgery deferred for days or weeks, the perioperative risks will be reduced.

Primary angioplasty

Background

Prior to the advent of thrombolysis or PTCA, the only means of achieving therapeutic reperfusion in patients with evolving MI was emergency CABG. Although no randomized trials have been performed, good results were reported for large case series from the 1970s, with an improvement in outcome compared to medically treated patients. Hospital mortality in the surgically treated patients was around 5 per cent, demonstrating that CABG can be performed in patients with evolving MI with an acceptable risk profile. With the advent of thrombolysis and primary PTCA, emergency CABG is now rarely performed in patients with evolving MI, unless there is an associated early mechanical complication such as a ventricular septal rupture or acute severe mitral regurgitation.

The use of primary PTCA to achieve reperfusion in evolving MI was first reported in 1983. Early case series suggested that primary PTCA was a safe and effective means of restoring antegrade flow in the infarct-related artery of a patient with evolving MI. Potential advantages compared to thrombolysis led to a series of randomized studies comparing primary PTCA with thrombolysis. To date, more than 4000 patients have been studied (with the largest trial being the recently reported DANAMI-2 study which randomized 1572 patients to primary PTCA or accelerated rt-PA). An overview of the short-term results suggests that:

- Primary PTCA is more effective at restoring adequate antegrade flow in the infarct related artery.
- Mortality is reduced by one-third with primary PTCA.
- Re-infarction is reduced by one-third with primary PTCA.
- Stroke is reduced by two-thirds with primary PTCA.

It is important to note that most of the individual trials were relatively small, different thrombolytic regimens were used, and patient selection criteria varied.

Long-term follow-up of some of the studies suggest that the early benefits are maintained for at least 5 years. The initial higher costs of primary PTCA are offset by cost savings associated with the prevention of complications. Most of the beneficial effect of primary PTCA is obtained when it is used in high risk patients (particularly those aged >70 years, with extensive myocardial infarction) and in those individuals who present several hours after the onset of symptoms (when the organized intracoronary thrombus has increased resistance to pharmacological lysis).

The randomized trials discussed above were performed in high volume expert centres. Data from large registries provide some information about the benefits of primary PTCA in clinical practice. In more than 30 000 patients enrolled in these observational studies, thrombolysis patients were treated more rapidly. Primary PTCA was most effective in patients treated early after hospital admission. There was no major reduction in mortality associated with primary PTCA. These data suggest that it may be difficult to replicate the results obtained in the randomized trials when primary PTCA is employed in routine clinical practice.

Selection of patients for primary angioplasty

Since less than 10 per cent of European hospitals have facilities for primary PTCA, thrombolysis will remain the best option for the treatment of evolving MI in most hospitals. When thrombolysis is contraindicated, recent studies suggest that patients can be safely transferred to interventional centres for primary PTCA with clinical benefit. In interventional centres, primary PTCA should be considered in preference to thrombolysis in higher risk patients. Patients who are likely to benefit most from primary PTCA are those with:

- age >70 years;
- ECG evidence of extensive MI;
- haemodynamic compromise [heart rate >100 b.p.m., or systolic blood pressure (BP) <100 mmHg].

A senior colleague should be contacted to discuss the choice of reperfusion strategy for these patients.

Antithrombotic therapy

Aspirin

Aspirin irreversibly inactivates platelet cyclooxygenase, reducing synthesis of thromboxane A2. This reduces platelet aggregation, enhancing recanalization in acute MI, and reducing the risk of further vascular events in patients with previous MI. The effect of aspirin on mortality in patients with acute MI has been studied in 15 trials, enrolling more than 19 000 patients (most of these patients were enrolled in ISIS-2). Overall mortality with aspirin therapy is reduced by around 20 per cent. This benefit is maintained with continued treatment over several years. A loading dose of 150 mg produces rapid and complete inhibition of thromboxane-mediated platelet inhibition. For long-term treatment, higher doses are more gastrotoxic. A dose of 75 mg/day maintains virtually complete long-term cyclooxygenase inhibition, and is suitable for chronic therapy.

There are few contraindications to the use of aspirin, but it should not be given to patients with:

- known hypersensitivity to aspirin;
- bleeding peptic ulcer;
- coagulation disorder;
- severe hepatic disease.

There is no clear evidence of a relationship between effectiveness and time from onset of symptoms, and aspirin should immediately be given to all patients diagnosed to have evolving or recent MI, even if presentation is late. If long-term therapy with aspirin is contraindicated or poorly tolerated, clopidogrel 75 mg daily is an alternative that has similar efficacy.

Anticoagulants

As previously discussed, heparin is required for 48 hours after thrombolysis with plasminogen activators. Heparin is not beneficial and is not recommended as routine therapy after streptokinase. If mobilization is delayed because of complications, the risk of deep vein thrombosis (DVT) and pulmonary embolism (PE) is increased, and patients should be treated with prophylactic subcutaneous heparin 5000 u b.d. The use of oral anticoagulants after MI has been studied in more than 30 000 patients. Compared with standard aspirin therapy, oral anticoagulation has no beneficial effects on adverse cardiac events, but it is associated with an increased bleeding risk. The combination of aspirin and oral anticoagulation may have some beneficial effects, but has not yet been evaluated in a sufficiently large series of trials. On the basis of these data, we recommend reserving oral anticoagulants for patients with a complication such as DVT, PE, atrial fibrillation (AF), thromboembolism or intracardiac thrombus.

Intravenous beta-blockers

Background

Beta-blockers have antiarrhythmic, anti-ischaemic and antihypertensive properties. Small studies indicate that these beneficial effects reduce chest pain, myocardial wall stress and infarct size in patients with MI. An overview of almost 30 000 patients randomized to placebo or intravenous therapy in the pre-thrombolytic era indicates that:

- They are well tolerated, with over 95 per cent of appropriately selected patients able to receive full IV doses of beta-blockers without significant adverse effects.
- They reduce early mortality (within the first 36 hours) by around 15 per cent. Subgroup analysis suggested that most of this mortality reduction is due to the prevention of cardiac rupture and VF and that mortality reduction is maximal in older patients with hypertension, a tachycardia or extensive infarction. Mortality reduction in low risk patients, who do not have any of these features, is minimal. In these trials, the number of lives saved by IV beta-blockers is similar to that observed for early non-selective angiotensin converting enzyme (ACE) inhibitor therapy in ISIS-4 and GISSI-3.
- They limit infarct size and preserve left ventricular function.

- They relieve ischaemic chest pain by reducing myocardial oxygen consumption.
- They reduce the incidence of ventricular and supraventricular arrhythmias by blocking the deleterious effects of catecholamines and suppressing automaticity.

Data relating to the combined use of thrombolysis and IV beta-blockers is limited. In the TIMI-IIB study, almost 1500 patients were randomized to receive IV beta-blockade or deferred oral therapy starting on day 6; IV beta-blockers were started shortly after thrombolytic therapy. The combination of thrombolytic therapy and IV beta-blockers was well tolerated, and was associated with a significant reduction in the incidence of early recurrent ischaemia, re-infarction and cerebral haemorrhage. There was no beneficial effect on mortality. On the basis of this data, IV beta-blocker therapy is not mandatory, but can be safely used in selected high risk patients.

Indications for IV beta-blocker therapy

Treatment with IV beta-blockers should be considered in all haemodynamically stable patients who present within 12 hours of the onset of symptoms of acute MI, with ST elevation in at least two leads, and who are free of contraindications. The groups of patients who will gain maximum benefit are:

- patients in whom thrombolytic therapy or PTCA are contraindicated or unavailable within 12 hours of the onset of symptoms;
- patients with continuing ischaemic chest pain following thrombolytic therapy and IV analgesia;
- patients at high risk of early complications (age >65 years, extensive or anterior infarction, resting sinus tachycardia, past history of ischaemic heart disease, diabetes mellitus or hypertension);
- patients who are hypertensive (systolic BP >160 mmHg), elderly or receive thrombolytic therapy relatively late, since these patients are at increased risk of early cardiac rupture.

Targeting IV beta-blocker therapy onto these four subgroups may help to maximize the gains from therapy, whilst limiting the number of patients who need to be treated. IV beta-blockers are preferable to nitrates for the control of peri-infarction hypertension (providing no contraindications are present), since they have additional beneficial effects on mortality.

Exclusion criteria for intravenous beta-blocker therapy

Patients are unsuitable for intravenous beta-blocker therapy if:

- the resting heart rate is below 60 b.p.m.;
- systolic blood pressure is below 100 mmHg;
- first, second or third degree heart block is present;
- bronchospasm is present on admission, or the patient has a history of airways disease;
- pre-treatment with a beta-blocker, diltiazem or verapamil has been given.

In patients with a marked resting tachycardia, it is important to exclude the presence of heart failure before administering IV beta-blockers.

Administration regimen for intravenous atenolol

Atenolol is useful for IV beta-blockade in acute MI, since its administration regimen is relatively simple. Atenolol is given by slow IV injection, followed by oral atenolol, with the dose adjusted to slow the heart rate. The administration regimen is as follows:

- 5 mg atenolol is given by slow IV injection over 5 minutes. This is stopped if the heart rate drops to 45 b.p.m. or below, systolic blood pressure drops to 100 mmHg or below, the PR interval is prolonged to more than 0.24 seconds or dyspnoea is aggravated.
- If heart rate remains above 60 b.p.m. 10 minutes after initial IV bolus of atenolol, a further IV injection of 2.5 mg is given, followed by a further 2.5 mg 2 minutes later (if necessary) to a maximum total dose of 10 mg over 6 minutes, observing the above cautions during each injection.
- Ten minutes after the end of the IV injection, 50 mg of oral atenolol is given if the heart rate >40 b.p.m.
- Long-term oral atenolol 50–100 mg daily is continued, unless a contraindication develops.

Adverse effects of intravenous beta-blocker therapy

Adverse effects of IV beta-blocker therapy are very rare, occurring in less than 5 per cent of patients treated. Precipitation of heart failure and heart block are the commonest important side effects, but are very rare in patients who have normal conduction and no evidence of heart failure.

When these complications do occur they are usually easily reversible, and are not associated with an adverse effect on prognosis. Specific adverse effects are treated as follows:

- Left ventricular failure should be treated by IV loop diuretics.
- Symptomatic sinus bradycardia or complete heart block should be treated with IV atropine 0.6 mg, repeated as necessary. In rare cases, an infusion of a beta-agonist (such as dobutamine or isoprenaline) or temporary pacing may be necessary.
- Hypotension should initially be treated with a dobutamine infusion. If hypotension is severe and prolonged, and is thought to be related to beta-blocker therapy, an infusion of glucagon (50 mg/kg as an IV bolus followed by an infusion of 1–5 mg per hour) will reverse the effects of the beta-receptor blockade by increasing intracellular cAMP levels.
- Bronchospasm may be precipitated in some susceptible individuals, and should be treated by withholding further doses of beta-blockers and treating the episode with nebulized beta-agonists.

Oral beta-blockers

Long-term oral beta-blockers, commenced in the convalescent phase of MI, have been evaluated in a large number of placebo-controlled trials. In a recent meta-analysis of 82 trials enrolling more than 54 000 patients, mortality was reduced by almost 25 per cent due to the prevention of re-infarction and sudden death. These benefits are apparent irrespective of age, site of infarction, and presence or absence of previous MI or complications. Serious side effects are rare. Benefit is still apparent after several years of therapy, and beta-blockers should therefore be continued indefinitely.

On the basis of these trial data, all patients should be considered for long-term oral beta-blocker therapy in the convalescent phase of MI. Contraindications to beta-blocker therapy are present in around 20 per cent of patients, and consist of:

- resting heart rate <60 b.p.m.;
- second or third degree heart block;
- a history of asthma, COPD or severe peripheral vascular disease.

Several different agents have been evaluated and shown to be effective.

Since side effects and compliance are problematic in some patients, a cardioselective agent is preferable. Treatment should be started between days 2 and 7, with an agent such as metoprolol 50 mg b.d., increased as necessary to obtain a resting heart rate of 50–60 b.p.m. and continued indefinitely. The maximum mortality benefit from beta-blocker therapy is obtained in higher risk patients, whose infarctions are complicated by arrhythmias or heart failure. These patients should initially be treated with appropriate antiarrhythmic and anti-failure therapy. Once their clinical condition is stabilized, a trial of beta-blocker therapy can be instituted. Treatment should be started with a low dose shorter-acting agent such as metoprolol 25 mg b.d., with the dose increased if tolerated.

Calcium channel blockers

Calcium channel blocking drugs have anti-ischaemic, vasodilating and antihypertensive properties that may be beneficial in patients with acute MI. A meta-analysis of more than 20 000 patients enrolled in placebo-controlled randomized trials, however, showed no significant beneficial effect on mortality. There is some evidence that the type of calcium antagonist used may be important. Dihydropyridine calcium antagonists are powerful vasodilators and may induce tachycardia, since they have no effect on the cardiac conduction system. In almost 10 000 studied patients dihydropyridine agents showed a trend towards increased mortality. Both diltiazem and verapamil have effects on the cardiac conduction system, slowing heart rate, potentially improving their efficacy in MI patients. In a series of trials randomizing 9000 patients (DAVIT-1, DAVIT-2, MDPIT and INTERCEPT), these drugs also had no significant beneficial effect on mortality, although the incidence of reinfarction and recurrent ischaemia was reduced. Subgroup analysis suggested that the overall neutral effect reflects an increase in mortality in patients with ventricular dysfunction, and a reduction in mortality in those with well preserved ventricular function.

These studies suggest that dihydropyridine calcium antagonists should be avoided in MI patients. Rate-slowing calcium antagonists such as verapamil and diltiazem should not be given to patients with important left ventricular dysfunction. For patients in whom a beta-blocker is contraindicated or poorly tolerated, and left ventricular function is well preserved, a rate-slowing calcium antagonist can be safely used for symptom control if required.

Left ventricular failure

Background

Left ventricular failure is common after MI. In patients with only a small area of infarction, catecholamine-mediated increase in heart rate and contractility in the normally functioning non-infarcted segments of left ventricle will prevent decompensation. In patients with more extensive infarction, those mechanisms are overwhelmed, left ventricular end diastolic pressure rises and pulmonary oedema occurs. In some patients, left ventricular failure is due to or exacerbated by infarct complications such as arrhythmia, severe mitral regurgitation or ventricular septal rupture. The occurrence of left ventricular failure is an adverse prognostic feature, with a close correlation between the degree of failure and mortality (with in-hospital mortality rising from 6 per cent in patients free of signs of left ventricular failure, to 38 per cent in those with extensive crepitations).

Diagnosis and assessment

Clinical diagnosis of left ventricular failure after MI is often difficult. Clinical signs, symptoms and investigational features are highly variable, inconsistent and only loosely correlated together. For example, basal crepitations are common in patients with lung disease, irrespective of the presence of left ventricular failure, and pronounced radiological pulmonary congestion can be present in a patient whose chest is clear to auscultation. Left ventricular failure should be suspected in any patient with MI and extensive ventricular dysfunction (due to a large MI, or a smaller MI occurring in a patient with previous ischaemic ventricular damage) who develops breathlessness in association with a third heart sound and crepitations. Physical signs can change rapidly, and the heart and lungs should be auscultated at regular intervals during the early phase of evolving MI. The chest x-ray may show abnormalities including cardiomegaly, upper lobe diversion and perihilar alveolar shadowing. If signs of left ventricular failure develop, a careful clinical assessment is required (including echocardiography if possible) to exclude a mechanical complication, such as severe acute mitral regurgitation or ventricular septal rupture.

Treatment

Treatment of left ventricular failure consists of measures to relieve distress, reduce cardiac filling pressures (by vasodilatation) and decrease intraventricular fluid volume (by induction of diuresis), leading to a fall in left ventricular end diastolic pressure with resolution of pulmonary oedema. Chronic drug therapy aims to prevent the recurrence of symptoms. In addition, in some patients left ventricular function will improve with resolution of myocardial stunning, helping to prevent recurrence of symptoms after the acute event. Treatment consists of:

- sitting the patient in an upright posture and giving oxygen. This helps to diminish venous return and improve oxygenation.
- giving diamorphine by slow IV injection in 2.0 mg boluses, along with an anti-emetic such as metoclopramide 10 mg. Diamorphine acts as a sedative to relieve distress, and as a vasodilator to improve pulmonary oedema.
- giving a loop diuretic such as frusemide 80–160 mg as a slow intravenous injection. Intravenous loop diuretics induce vasodilatation followed by diuresis, improving left ventricular failure by a dual mechanism of action.
- if blood pressure is adequate (>100 mmHg), commencing an intravenous nitrate infusion as detailed in Appendix A. Nitrate-induced vasodilatation helps to reduce venous return, leading to a fall in left ventricular end diastolic pressure and an improvement in pulmonary oedema. The nitrate infusion should commence at a low dose, increased periodically. The dose should be titrated to produce a fall in BP of 15 mmHg, if possible, although BP should not be allowed to fall below 100 mmHg.

If these measures fail to control the situation, a further IV bolus of frusemide should be given and a senior colleague consulted. If a surgically treatable infarct-related complication can be identified, such as acute severe mitral regurgitation or ventricular septal rupture, insertion of an intra-aortic balloon pump or assisted ventilation (which can be instituted non-invasively using mask-based systems) may help to stabilize the patient for long enough to allow corrective surgery. In the absence of a treatable complication, the prognosis of severe left ventricular failure that does not respond to diamorphine, diuretics and nitrates is poor.

Cardiogenic shock

Background

Cardiogenic shock occurs in 5–10 per cent of patients with acute MI, and is responsible for the majority of in-hospital deaths. There has been no reduction in the incidence of cardiogenic shock since the widespread introduction of thrombolysis. Cardiogenic shock complicating acute MI can be due to:

- infarction or ischaemia of >40 per cent of the left ventricular myocardium leading to pump failure (85 per cent of cases);
- a potentially reversible complication leading to severe decompensation, such as acute mitral regurgitation, ventricular septal rupture or right ventricular infarction (15 per cent of cases).

In patients who present with an extensive infarction, cardiogenic shock usually develops early (within 24 hours of admission). If cardiogenic shock develops later, a careful assessment of the patient is required. In this situation cardiogenic shock is often associated with recurrent ischaemia leading to infarct extension and further impairment of left ventricular function, or to a mechanical complication, which may be amenable to surgical correction. Data from registry studies of cardiogenic shock treated by medical therapy suggest that mortality remains around 80–90 per cent. The factors associated with an increased risk of developing cardiogenic shock are:

- extensive Q wave anterior MI, MI associated with left bundle branch block, or failure of reperfusion;
- MI occurring in patients with previous infarction or CABG;
- increasing age or female sex;
- hypertension;
- diabetes.

Treatment in cardiogenic shock is designed to improve myocardial perfusion and function by administering inotropes, use of intra-aortic balloon counterpulsation and emergency revascularization. Data derived from case series, registry studies and retrospective analysis of thrombolysis trial databases suggest that early aggressive supportive therapy combined with cardiac catheterization and revascularization may favourably influence mortality. Stabilization and revascularization may be beneficial by aiding recovery of stunned myocardium around the edge of the infarct zone, allowing some recovery and improvement in myocardial function. These studies are compromised by their non-randomized trial design, and the potential confounding effect of patient selection bias, which may skew the results in favour of revascularization (since the fittest youngest patients who are most likely to survive are the cases most likely to undergo intensive treatment and revascularization). Randomized trials have been difficult to organize, but some information is now available. The Swiss Multicentre trial of Angioplasty for Shock (SMASH) demonstrated that revascularization was associated with a nonsignificant trend to reduced mortality although the small size of the study (55 patients) did not allow a statistically reliable conclusion to be reached. The SHould we emergently revascularize Occluded Coronaries for shocK (SHOCK) trial randomized 302 patients to receive either early revascularization or medical therapy. Survival was non-significantly improved at 30 days, and significantly improved at 6 months (50.3 per cent mortality in the revascularization group compared with 63.1 per cent mortality with medical therapy). Subgroup analysis suggested a larger benefit for younger (<75 years of age) patients treated early (within 6 hours of diagnosis). Taken together, this body of non-randomized and randomized trial data suggests that selected patients with cardiogenic shock may benefit from intensive supportive therapy combined with revascularization.

Diagnosis

A diagnosis of cardiogenic shock due to left ventricular dysfunction can be confidently made in patients with evidence of extensive ischaemic myocardial damage who present within 24 hours of the onset of an acute MI with features of:

- hypotension (systolic BP persistently <90 mmHg);
- clinical signs of a low output sate (urine output <30 mL/h, poor peripheral perfusion or impaired cerebration);
- evidence of raised cardiac filling pressures (the presence of clinical or radiological pulmonary oedema implies that pulmonary artery wedge pressure is >15 mmHg).

If there are atypical features to the clinical presentation, careful evaluation is required to exclude treatable complications of MI. In particular, if there is:

- late onset of cardiogenic shock or an associated new murmur, the cardiogenic shock may be due to a mechanical complication;
- low blood pressure in the absence of pulmonary oedema in a patient with inferior or posterior infarction or a negative fluid balance, when hypotension may be due to right ventricular infarction or hypovolaemia.

If any doubt exists as to the cause of the cardiogenic shock, echocardiography and pulmonary artery catheterization are required. In patients with cardiogenic shock due to severe left ventricular dysfunction there will be extensive left ventricular hypokinesia at echocardiography in association with a raised (>15 mmHg) pulmonary wedge pressure and a low (<2.2 L/min/m^2) cardiac index.

Management of cardiogenic shock due to severe ischaemic left ventricular dysfunction

In treating these patients, the priorities are to stabilize the haemo-dynamic situation, and identify patients who are likely to benefit from aggressive intervention. Stabilizing the haemodynamic state requires:

- treatment of arrhythmias;
- giving oxygen for hypoxia;
- treating pulmonary oedema with intravenous frusemide;
- commencing a dobutamine infusion (5–20 μg/kg/min) to attempt to increase cardiac output;
- commencing a dopamine infusion (2.5–5.0 μg/kg/min via a central line) to increase renal blood flow.

In a patient less than 75 years of age who has presented early, cardiac catheterization and (if possible) PTCA should be considered. Patients unsuitable for revascularization, or those who show a poor haemody-namic response to inotropes (with a blood pressure that dose not rise to >100 mmHg) have a very poor prognosis and are not likely to survive. If an underlying mechanical complication such as ventricular septal rupture or acute severe mitral regurgitation is present, and surgical correction is possible, insertion of an intra-aortic balloon pump or ven-tilation should be considered to help stabilize the patient.

Management of hypotension associated with right ventricular infarction or hypovolaemia

Right ventricular infarction commonly occurs in association with an extensive infero-posterior MI due to proximal occlusion of a large right coronary artery. Ischaemic damage leads to a rise in right ventricular end diastolic pressure and reduction in right ventricular stroke volume. The infarcted dilated right ventricle impairs left ventricular filling. These two mechanisms lead to a fall in cardiac output and systemic hypotension. Atrial fibrillation and complete heart block occur in about a third of patients with right ventricular infarction. These arrhythmias cause fur-ther haemodynamic deterioration due to loss of atrial transport in a situ-ation where ventricular filling is already compromised. Right ventricular infarction should be suspected in any patient with inferior infarction who develops hypotension. The diagnosis can be confirmed by:

- the presence of hypotension in association with a raised jugular venous pressure (JVP) and clear lung fields;

- ST elevation in a V4R lead;
- insertion of a pulmonary artery catheter and echocardiography.

Patients with right ventricular infarction as the cause of their hypotension have a characteristic haemodynamic profile, with a low or normal wedge pressure in association with a raised right ventricular diastolic and right atrial pressure. Echocardiography is required to ensure that the hypotension is not due to a ventricular septal rupture or acute severe mitral regurgitation.

Improving outcome in patients with right ventricular infarction depends on increasing right ventricular preload by fluid loading and avoiding vasodilator drugs, correcting arrhythmias and using inotropes only when fluid balance has been optimized. Treatment therefore consists of:

- insertion of a pulmonary artery catheter to confirm diagnosis and guide treatment;
- avoiding treatment with diuretics or vasodilators, which will exacerbate the haemodynamic problem by reducing preload;
- fluid loading with 200 mL physiological saline over 10 minutes, following by 1–2 litres over 2–4 hours, followed by 200 mL/h. The infusion rate should be carefully titrated to maintain an optimal wedge pressure of 15 mmHg.
- if hypotension persists despite an optimal wedge pressure, treating with intravenous inotropes;
- if complete heart block occurs, restoring AV synchrony with temporary dual chamber pacing;
- if AF occurs, restoring AV synchrony with cardioversion.

With aggressive treatment, mortality in hypotensive patients with right ventricular infarction can be reduced to 20–30 per cent.

If fluid intake is poor or aggressive diuretic therapy has been employed, hypotension can occur in the absence of major left or right ventricular dysfunction, due to intravascular volume depletion. These patients will have hypotension, clear lung fields and a normal venous pressure. A V4R recording will normally show no ST elevation. It can be difficult to confidently differentiate this from right ventricular infarction, and a pulmonary artery catheter will be required to clarify the diagnosis and guide therapy. In patients with intravascular volume depletion, wedge pressure, right ventricular and right atrial pressures will be low. Treatment consists of withholding diuretics and vasodilators and expanding intravascular volume with intravenous fluids.

ACE inhibitors

Background

Activation of the renin–angiotensin system is an early compensatory response to an evolving MI. Activation of the renin–angiotensin system leads to vasoconstriction, increased heart rate and sympathetic activation. In the early phases of evolving MI these deleterious changes will increase ventricular wall stress, increase oxygen consumption and reduce electrical stability. In the longer term, persistent activation of the renin–angiotensin system potentiates adverse remodelling, leading to ventricular dilatation and heart failure. The adverse consequences of renin–angiotensin activation can be blocked by the use of ACE inhibitors with potentially beneficial effects on mortality. More than 100 000 patients have been evaluated in a series of trials that reported in the 1990s (GISSI-3, ISIS-4, AIRE, SAVE, CCS-1 and TRACE). Trials of short-term non-selective ACE inhibitor therapy started early after MI demonstrated a small (approximately 6.5 per cent) reduction in 30-day mortality with treatment. Trials of long-term selective therapy in high risk patients (with clinical evidence of heart failure or evidence of substantial left ventricular dysfunction) demonstrated a large (approximately 20 per cent) reduction in mortality, with particular benefit in diabetics (in keeping with the recently reported HOPE study). Importantly, ACE inhibitor therapy was generally well tolerated. On the basis of these trial data, ACE inhibitors should be prescribed early after MI in patients who are clinically stable with an adequate blood pressure. If possible, treatment should be initiated within 24 hours of admission, titrated up to target doses, and continued for at least 30 days. In high risk patients (those with clinical evidence of heart failure, a large MI, evidence of substantial impairment of left ventricular function or diabetes), ACE inhibitor therapy should be continued indefinitely. In low risk patients (small uncomplicated MI, well preserved left ventricular function, no diabetes), long-term ACE inhibitor therapy is not mandatory.

Patient selection and drug administration

All patients who are clinically stable should be assessed with a view to initiating ACE inhibitor therapy early after MI. The major contraindications to therapy early after MI are:

- hypotension (supine blood pressure <100 mmHg).
- significant valve stenosis;

- history of angio-oedema or prior allergy to ACE inhibitors;
- renal impairment.

Several drugs have been evaluated in post-MI trials. Treatment should be initiated with a small test dose of one of the proven drugs. The recommended test doses are:

- captopril 6.25 mg
- lisinopril 5 mg
- ramipril 2.5 mg
- trandolapril 0.5 mg.

Blood pressure should be monitored hourly after the test dose. If the test dose is well tolerated after 12 hours (systolic blood pressure remains above 100 mmHg), chronic therapy can be initiated, and the dose escalated daily, aiming to achieve a target level (50 mg tds of captopril, 10 mg once daily of lisinopril, 5 mg b.d. of ramipril or 4 mg once daily of trandolapril) if dose increments are tolerated. Renal function and electrolytes should be monitored to ensure there is no ACE inhibitor induced deterioration in renal function.

Treatment policy should be reviewed when the patient is seen for follow-up. In high risk patients it is important to ensure that dosage is increased to target levels if possible. In low risk patients, ACE inhibitor therapy can be discontinued after a minimum of 30 days of treatment provided there is no other indication to continue the drug.

Mechanical complications

Ventricular free wall rupture

Rupture of the free wall of the left ventricle occurs in up to 3 per cent of all hospitalized patients with MI, accounting for 20 per cent of hospital deaths. Risk factors for free wall rupture are:

- increasing age
- female sex
- first infarct
- hypertension
- marked/persistent ST elevation.

In addition, the incidence of free wall rupture may be increased by thrombolytic therapy, particularly if it is given late in the course of the infarct. Intravenous beta-blocker therapy reduces the risk of free wall rupture. Free wall ruptures present within a few days of the onset of MI. The usual presentation is with a sudden acute rupture presenting as collapse with electromechanical dissociation which does not respond to resuscitation. In 25 per cent of cases a subacute rupture occurs, with a slower leak of blood into the pericardial space producing tamponade.

Echocardiography confirms the presence of fluid in the pericardial space. Immediate surgery should be considered, as there is a high risk of major rupture and death occurring unpredictably.

Ventricular septal rupture

Ventricular septal rupture occurs in up to 2 per cent of hospitalized patients with MI, with most cases occurring within the first post-infarct week. With anterior infarction, the defect is usually apical and involves one direct perforation. With inferior infarction, the defect is often a complex serpiginous or fenestrated lesion involving the posterior or basal septum; these complex defects are more technically difficult to surgically repair. Patients present with signs and symptoms of heart failure in association with a new pansystolic murmur, maximal at the lower left sternal edge. The clinical presentation may be confusing, with progression to cardiogenic shock and a minimal murmur. The diagnosis can be confirmed by echocardiography or right heart catheterization. The diagnostic features are:

- visible defect in intraventricular septum with jet crossing from left to right ventricle on echocardiography;
- an increase in oxygen saturation from right atrium to right ventricle of >10 per cent due to oxygenated blood crossing the septum via the defect. A large increase in saturation implies the presence of a large defect.

When the diagnosis has been established, supportive therapy with diuretics, nitrates, inotropes and an intra-aortic balloon pump may help to stabilize the haemodynamic status. Without corrective surgery, 90 per cent of patients die, usually within days of diagnosis. Even with surgery, mortality is 25–50 per cent (with mortality risk increased in older patients, those with major haemodynamic compromise, and when the defect complicates inferior infarction). Surgery should probably be carried out as early as possible, since most patients will develop progressive haemodynamic compromise with multi-organ failure if the operation is delayed, and this decreases the chance of surviving an operation.

Acute mitral regurgitation

A mild degree of mitral regurgitation occurs in 40 per cent of patients with MI. This mild regurgitation is related to ventricular dilatation and shape change (which distort mitral annulus geometry) or papillary muscle dysfunction (which interferes with mitral leaflet function). The postero-medial papillary muscle is more vulnerable to ischaemia since its blood supply is derived solely from the circumflex artery, whereas the antero-lateral papillary muscle has a dual vascular supply (from the circumflex and left anterior descending). This mild degree of mitral regurgitation is usually well tolerated, and detectable only by the presence of a mitral pansystolic murmur. The mitral regurgitant murmur may be transitory, disappearing as reperfusion or recovery of left ventricular function restores mitral annulus geometry or papillary muscle function.

Severe acute mitral regurgitation complicates around 1 per cent of patients with MI, usually early in the first post-infarct week. The mechanism is usually rupture of the postero-medial papillary muscle complicating an inferior MI, leading to a flail posterior mitral leaflet. Severe acute mitral regurgitation can occur as a consequence of a small localized sub-endocardial infarct in a patient with well preserved left ventricular function if the area of infarction involves the postero-medial papillary muscle. Patients present with severe heart failure, which may progress to cardiogenic shock. There may be a new loud pansystolic murmur, maximal at the apex and radiating to the axilla. If the pressure gradient between the left ventricle and left atrium is minimal (due to pressure equalization between the two chambers when the regurgitation is severe), the murmur may be minimal or absent. Even in the absence of a characteristic murmur, acute severe mitral regurgitation should be looked for in any patient who develops severe heart failure, particularly if the onset is delayed or the deterioration occurs in a patient with inferior infarction with preserved left ventricular function.

Patients with suspected acute severe mitral regurgitation require urgent evaluation with a view to emergency surgery. The diagnosis can be confirmed by:

- echocardiography; this may show a flail leaflet and doppler evidence of severe mitral regurgitation. The left atrium is often not enlarged.
- right heart catheterization and oximetry; oximetry shows no shunt, and prominent V waves may be visible in the pulmonary artery wedge pressure trace.

Treatment with diuretics, vasodilators and an intra-aortic balloon pump may help to stabilize the patient initially, but mortality without operation is >90 per cent. Urgent mitral valve surgery is required for all suitable patients. Perioperative mortality is 30 per cent and patients who survive to discharge have a good long-term prognosis.

Early peri-infarction arrhythmias

Background

Peri-infarction arrhythmias (occurring within 48 hours) are very common in patients with acute MI, and are an important cause of death. Acute myocardial ischaemia induces a wide range of detrimental changes in myocyte metabolism (intracellular acidosis, raised cAMP, raised sodium, magnesium and calcium). These occur in association with adverse changes in systemic biochemical and physiological function induced by the evolving infarct (systemic acidosis, abnormal potassium, lactate, adenosine, CO_2 and lysophospho-glycerides along with catecholamine release and autonomic disturbance). These factors interact to destabilize myocardial electrical function, leading to the induction of peri-infarction arrhythmias. Even a small area of ischaemia or infarction can develop electrical instability, leading to the induction of potentially lethal arrhythmias. These local and systemic proarrhythmic disturbances are maximal early after the onset of MI, resolving within 48 hours, thereby reducing the risk of late arrhythmia recurrence due to these mechanisms. Since these early peri-infarction arrhythmias are not related to infarct size and have a low recurrence rate, they are not invariably associated with a poor long-term prognosis.

Infarct site has an important influence on the type of peri-infarction arrhythmias that occur. In patients with anterior infarction there is a relative excess of sympathetic activation, promoting the induction of tachyarrhythmias in areas of enhanced automaticity. There is a high density of vagal receptors in the infero-posterior wall of the left ventricle, which are activated during inferior infarction. The resultant increase in vagal activity, acting in conjunction with infarct-related disturbance of function in the conduction system, increases the incidence of bradyarrhythmias.

Supraventricular and ventricular ectopic beats

Frequent ectopic beats occur in the majority of patients with evolving MI. Supraventricular ectopic beats are due to enhanced automaticity in the atria or AV junction. Since ventricular activation occurs via the normal conduction system, supraventricular ectopics are characterized by a

QRS complex of normal morphology, which occurs prematurely and may be preceded by an abnormal P wave. Ventricular ectopics arise due to enhanced automaticity in the ventricular myocardium. Since depolarization occurs outside the normal conduction system, the resultant QRS complex has a broad configuration. Ectopic beats are usually asymptomatic, and are not associated with an adverse prognosis, regardless of their frequency and complexity. When frequent ectopics occur:

- pain relief should be adequate – if continuing ischaemic pain is present, use of IV beta-blockade or further diamorphine should be considered;
- heart failure should be looked for and treated if present;
- electrolytes should be checked and oral supplements given if potassium is <4.0 mmol/L.
- giving intravenous magnesium should be considered if the patient has been on long-term diuretic therapy prior to admission.

There is no evidence that suppression of ectopics with antiarrhythmic drugs prevents the occurrence of life-threatening arrhythmias or improves prognosis.

Sinus tachycardia

Sinus tachycardia is common after an acute MI, and is often associated with extensive anterior infarction, sympathetic activation and an adverse prognosis. In sinus tachycardia, each QRS complex is preceded by a normal P wave, the QRS complexes are of normal morphology, and the rate is normally less than 140 b.p.m. If sinus tachycardia is persistent and excessive, it may cause extension of myocardial necrosis by increasing oxygen consumption. If sinus tachycardia is persistent:

- adequate analgesia should be ensured;
- heart failure should be looked for and treated;
- beta-blockade should be considered if there are no contraindications.

Prolonged sinus tachycardia is most likely to occur in a patient with extensive infarction and major left ventricular impairment.

Atrial tachyarrhythmias

Peri-infarction AF occurs in 10–20 per cent of patients. Atrial electrical instability or stretch leads to the development of multiple micro re-entry circuits within the atrium leading to chaotic atrial electrical activity which is intermittently conducted via the AV node to erratically depolarize the ventricles. The rapid ventricular rate and loss of AV synchrony results in a significant reduction in cardiac output and an increase in ischaemia. Characteristic ECG features of AF are an irregular baseline due to fibrillation waves (often best seen in V1) with completely irregular ventricular activity. The incidence of AF is increased in patients with:

- large infarctions
- increased age
- pericarditis
- right ventricular infarction
- diabetes
- hypertension
- inotrope use.

The development of early (<24 hours) AF is usually associated with inferior infarction, whilst later (>24 hours) AF is usually associated with anterior infarction and heart failure. Mortality is more than doubled in MI patients who develop AF.

The treatment of peri-infarction AF depends on the ventricular rate and associated clinical features:

- If the ventricular rate is rapid (>200 b.p.m.), systolic BP is low (<90 mmHg) or the arrhythmia is associated with chest pain, heart failure or impaired consciousness, immediate direct current cardioversion (DCC) is the treatment of choice.
- Many episodes of post-infarction AF are short-lived (50 per cent last less than 30 minutes) and well tolerated. If AF occurs with a rate of <110 b.p.m., systolic blood pressure is maintained above 90 mmHg and there are no associated symptoms, no treatment is necessary initially.
- If AF persists for more than 30 minutes, has a rate consistently >110 b.p.m., is associated with a fall in systolic BP or with rate-related symptoms, drug treatment is indicated.

A variety of drugs can be used to treat patients with peri-infarction AF. In patients with coexistent symptomatic left ventricular dysfunction, digoxin (0.25–0.5 mg IV every 6–8 hours up to a maximum of 1 mg/24 hours) helps to slow ventricular rate and its inotropic properties may improve cardiac function. Digoxin slows ventricular rate by an indirect effect on AV nodal conduction, mediated by an increase in parasympathetic activity. In patients with acute infarction who have extensive sympathetic activation and vagal inhibition, this mechanism may be relatively ineffective. In patients who have no signs of heart failure (or other contraindication), intravenous atenolol is effective for rapid ventricular rate control. If a central venous line is in place, intravenous amiodarone is useful. This can be administered to patients regardless of left ventricular function. In addition to achieving rapid ventricular rate control (due to a beta-blocking effect) amiodarone also has a beneficial effect on atrial electrical stability. This helps to restore sinus rhythm in up to 75 per cent of treated patients within 4 hours. If it is important to restore sinus rhythm and a central line is not *in situ*, IV amiodarone can be given via a large-bore peripheral cannula, provided the infusion is used for a maximum of 24 hours (see Appendix A).

All patients with AF should be anticoagulated with heparin. If the arrhythmia persists for more than 24 hours, restoration of sinus rhythm by electrical cardioversion should be considered to reduce the long-term risk of arrhythmia-associated thromboembolism. Atrial flutter is less common than AF, but presents and is managed in a similar fashion.

Idioventricular rhythm

Idioventricular rhythym is a very common peri-infarction arrhythmia, presenting as a regular broad complex tachycardia with a stable QRS configuration and a rate of less than 120 b.p.m. It is due to enhanced automaticity in a ventricular focus, and is often associated with spontaneous or therapeutic reperfusion. Idioventricular rhythm is rarely associated with haemodynamic compromise and has no adverse effect on mortality. Since the arrhythmia is usually well tolerated, no specific treatment is required.

Ventricular tachycardia

Non-sustained VT (three or more consecutive ventricular beats at a rate >120 b.p.m., lasting for less than 30 seconds) occurs in up to 7 per cent of peri-infarct patients. When it occurs in patients with previous MI or has a rapid rate, it may be a marker of an adverse prognosis. In most patients it is asymptomatic, and antiarrhythmic therapy (with the exception of beta-blockers) should be avoided. As for other non-sustained peri-infarction arrhythmias, treatment should be directed towards control of pain, ongoing cardiac ischaemia, heart failure and correction of electrolyte disturbance. If episodes of non-sustained VT are frequent, prolonged or symptomatic, and do not respond to the above measures, the use of a lignocaine infusion should be considered.

Sustained VT (lasting for >30 seconds) is relatively uncommon, occurring in up to 2 per cent of post-infarct patients. The occurrence of sustained

VT is associated with extensive ventricular dysfunction and recurrent ischaemia, and is therefore a marker of increased hospital mortality. Monomorphic VT presents as a regular broad complex tachycardia with a rate >120 b.p.m. Polymorphic VT presents as a broad complex tachycardia with variable morphology. Polymorphic VT is usually rapid and poorly tolerated. Sustained VT has important adverse effects in post-infarct patients, leading to:

- hypotension and heart failure if the ventricular rate is rapid and left ventricular function poor;
- ischaemia and infarct extension due to increased myocardial oxygen consumption;
- further electrical instability (exacerbated by the above mechanisms) leading to VF.

The onset of sustained VT is therefore a medical emergency. Treatment selection depends on the degree of haemodynamic compromise that occurs:

- If systolic BP <90 mmHg or the patient has chest pain, a reduced conscious level or heart failure related to the tachycardia, DC cardioversion is the treatment of choice. If consciousness is lost with the onset of VT, the shock should be administered immediately. If the patient remains conscious, despite haemodynamic compromise, sedation with 2–10 mg IV midazolam is given prior to cardioversion.
- If systolic BP >90 mmHg and the patient is not distressed or poorly perfused, initial treatment should be with lignocaine 50 mg IV over 2 minutes, repeated every 5 minutes if the arrhythmia does not terminate, to a maximum dose of 200 mg. Lignocaine is preferable to other class 1 agents since its vasoconstrictor properties limit the occurrence of drug-induced hypotension, and its initial short half-life enables other antiarrhythmic agents to be administered if it is initially ineffective without an excessive risk of drug interaction. Lignocaine has only limited efficacy, and often fails to terminate VT.
- If the lignocaine bolus terminates the VT, an infusion of 500 mg lignocaine in 500 mL of 5 per cent dextrose at an infusion rate of 4 mg/min for 30 minutes, 2 mg/min for 2 hours and 1 mg/min for 24 hours should be commenced. Since lignocaine is metabolized in the liver, the infusion rate in patients with liver disease or impaired hepatic perfusion due to heart failure should be reduced. Electrolytes and blood gases should be checked and clinical evidence of heart failure sought. Failure is treated with diuretics or nitrates, and oxygen given if hypoxia is present. If serum potassium is less than 4.0 mmol/L, potassium supplements are given IV.

- If VT recurs despite the lignocaine infusion, a further bolus of 100 mg lignocaine is given, the infusion rate is increased to 2 mg/min for 1 hour, and IV magnesium given. The 12-lead ECG is checked to ensure QT interval is not prolonged; if QT > 420 milliseconds, further antiarrhythmic drug therapy should not be given and a senior colleague should be consulted, as pacing therapy may help to shorten the QT and suppress the arrhythmia.
- If the VT is not terminated by the initial bolus of 200 mg lignocaine, or recurs despite an infusion and further boluses of lignocaine plus administration of potassium and magnesium and the patient remains haemodynamically stable, amiodarone has demonstrated the ability to suppress VT resistant to class 1 agents in many patients. The 12-lead ECG should be checked to ensure QT interval is not prolonged. Treatment with lignocaine should be discontinued and amiodarone given IV (see Appendix A).
- If VT persists and the patient deteriorates haemodynamically during lignocaine or amiodarone administration, immediate DCC should be performed. If both lignocaine and amiodarone fail to terminate the VT, further drug therapy is contraindicated, as administration of multiple antiarrhythmics will increase the risk of adverse effects. The amiodarone infusion should be continued and DCC performed if required. Temporary overdrive pacing may be effective in terminating episodes of drug-resistant VT. A pacing lead should be inserted into the right ventricle. When VT occurs, pacing therapy should be instituted at a rate 20 per cent faster than the VT for 10 seconds, then abruptly discontinued. If the pacing therapy is successful, sinus rhythm will return. The ECG should be checked and pacing instituted if the QT interval is prolonged. Rapid VT or VF may be precipitated by overdrive pacing, requiring immediate cardioversion. The addition of high dose beta-blockade, and haemodynamic support with a balloon pump may also help to suppress the arrhythmia.

Since these arrhythmias are often associated with left ventricular impairment or recurrent ischaemia, treatment with diuretics, nitrates and anti-ischaemic agents should be optimized, and early cardiac catheterization considered.

Ventricular fibrillation

Ventricular fibrillation is characterized by rapid disorganized multiple re-entrant wavelets in the ventricle, resulting in loss of co-ordinated ventricular myocyte activity with loss of output and cardiac arrest. Untreated the arrhythmia is fatal, and is responsible for most pre-hospital deaths in patients with evolving MI. Most episodes occur early, with 80 per cent occurring within 12 hours of symptom onset. If defibrillation is performed rapidly, most episodes of VF can be reversed, but success rate declines rapidly with time. When VF occurs early in patients with good left ventricular function, long-term survival is not compromised; when VF occurs late in patients with heart failure, it is often a terminal event. The protocol for treatment of VF is detailed in Chapter 3.

Sinus bradycardia

Sinus bradycardia (<60 b.p.m.) is common early after acute MI, particularly in patients with inferior infarction and vagal activation. If the heart rate is persistently below 45 b.p.m. or there are rate-related symptoms, a bolus of atropine 0.6 mg IV (repeated as necessary) will increase the sinus rate. If sinus bradycardia persists despite repeated boluses of atropine, temporary pacing should be considered.

Conduction disturbances in relation to infarct site

A variety of conduction disturbances can occur in patients with evolving MI. Although early reperfusion with thrombolysis has shortened the duration of symptomatic episodes and reduced the need for temporary pacing, the incidence of AV block has remained relatively constant. When a conduction disturbance occurs in a patient with inferior infarction, it is usually due to vagal activation, AV nodal ischaemia, or both. If complete heart block develops, it is usually well tolerated. Since there is no damage to the conduction system in the ventricles, a secondary pacemaker in the bundle of His takes over ventricular activation, producing a stable reliable rhythm with a rate of >40 b.p.m., which is usually sufficient to maintain the circulation with no compromise. This escape rhythm is conducted via the normal ventricular activation pathways, and therefore will have a narrow QRS configuration. Normal AV nodal function recovers within hours or days, with a return to normal sinus rhythm.

By contrast, when AV block develops in a patient with anterior infarction, it is often poorly tolerated and is associated with a high risk of early death. For AV block to occur in anterior infarction, extensive and widespread damage to the left ventricular myocardium and the interventricular septum must occur, and the patients often die from heart failure. In these patients, the conduction disturbance is related to infarction of the bundle of His within the interventricular septum. The secondary pacemaker that is responsible for ventricular activation will be situated outside the specialized conduction system in the surviving ventricular myocardium. The escape rhythm generated by this type of secondary pacemaker will often have an unreliable rate of <40 b.p.m. (since the inherent automaticity of cells outside the specialized conduction system is usually low), and will have a broad QRS configuration as ventricular activation will be slow. This slow rate will be poorly tolerated in a patient with extensive ventricular damage, and episodes of unpredictable ventricular asystole often occur. When AV block occurs following acute anterior infarction, temporary pacing is usually required. If the patient survives the acute episode, the AV block is often persistent or recurrent, and a permanent pacemaker may be required.

In extensive anterior infarction with involvement of the septum, ischaemic damage to the bundle of His may lead to left or right bundle branch block on the surface EGG. The development of left bundle branch block usually indicates that extensive myocardial necrosis has occurred, with associated significant left ventricular dysfunction and a poor prognosis. Right bundle branch block can occur with less extensive infarction, as can involvement of only the anterior fascicle of the left bundle, leading to left axis deviation. Patients who develop left bundle branch block in combination with a long PR interval, or the combination of right bundle branch block, left axis deviation and a long PR interval, have suffered extensive damage to their conduction system; such patients should be discussed with a senior colleague, as prophylactic temporary pacing may be indicated to avert the need for pacemaker insertion in a compromised patient if sudden complete heart block with a slow escape rhythm develops.

First degree heart block

First degree AV block manifests with prolongation of the PR interval (Figure 1.5). It is the most common conduction disturbance, occurring in up to 15 per cent of patients, usually associated with inferior infarction. Progression to self-terminating and well tolerated episodes of high grade AV block is common. No specific treatment is required, other than withholding drugs (such as beta-blockers or digoxin), which impair AV nodal conduction, and closely monitoring the patient.

Mobitz type I (Wenckebach) heart block

Mobitz type I block is common after inferior infarction. It often occurs in patients who progress from first degree, through Mobitz type I to

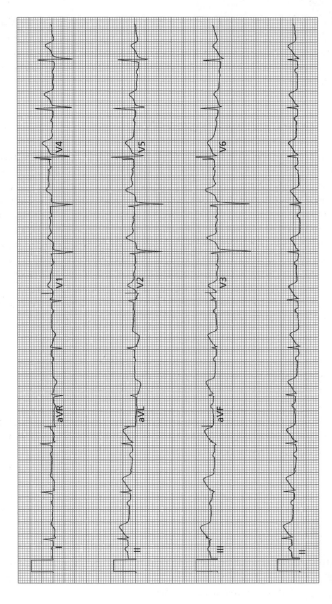

Figure 1.5 Acute inferior myocardial infarction with first degree AV block.

well tolerated complete block with a narrow complex escape rhythm. The ECG shows a progressive increase in PR interval culminating in a complete failure of conduction and a dropped beat. Apart from avoiding AV nodal blocking drugs, no treatment other than close observation is required.

Mobitz type II second degree block

Mobitz type II block is less common, and manifests itself as sudden unpredictable failure of AV nodal conduction, resulting in a dropped beat with no preceding change in the PR interval. Mobitz type II block is usually associated with septal involvement in extensive anterior infarction, leading to ischaemic damage to the bundle of His, and often coexists with bundle branch block. Mobitz type II block frequently progresses to poorly tolerated complete heart block with a slow and unreliable broad complex escape rhythm. Patients with anterior infarction who develop Mobitz type II block have a poor prognosis. When Mobitz type II block occurs, a senior colleague should be consulted, as prophylactic temporary pacing may be indicated to avert the need for pacemaker insertion in a compromised patient if sudden complete heart block with a slow escape rhythm develops.

Third degree (complete) heart block

Complete heart block occurs in up to 6 per cent of infarcts, and presents with complete dissociation between atrial and ventricular activity (Figure 1.6). The pathophysiology and recommended treatment depend on the site of infarction associated with the heart block.

In inferior infarction, patients usually progress through first degree and Wenckebach block to well tolerated complete heart block with a narrow complex escape rhythm. If the blood pressure is well maintained and the patient is asymptomatic, no treatment is necessary. If the ventricular rate falls below 40 b.p.m., pauses of >3 seconds occur, the systolic BP falls below 90 mmHg or rate-related symptoms develop:

- atropine 0.6 mg should be given intravenously, repeated as necessary.
- if symptomatic complete heart block persists despite atropine, a temporary pacing wire should be inserted.

Normal AV nodal conduction usually returns within 48 hours, a permanent pacemaker is not required, and prognosis after discharge from hospital is good.

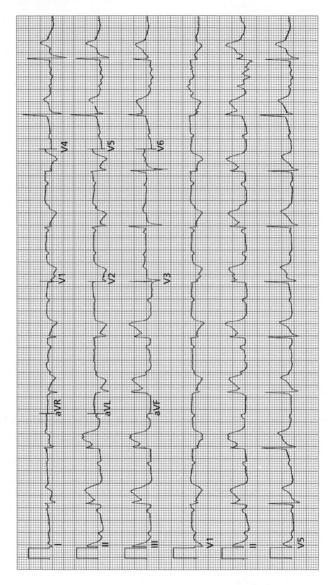

Figure 1.6 Acute inferior myocardial infarction with complete AV block.

In patients with anterior infarction, complete heart block often occurs suddenly, particularly in patients who develop left bundle branch block or have a period of Mobitz type II block. The escape rhythm is broad complex and slow, often associated with severe haemodynamic compromise in a patient with extensive infarction and major left ventricular impairment. Temporary pacing is always required to maintain an adequate rate. High grade AV block often persists, necessitating permanent pacemaker implantation. A large proportion of patients who develop complete heart block following anterior infarction die, often from pump failure due to ventricular damage.

Permanent cardiac pacing after MI

In patients with inferior MI, high degree AV block is usually self-limiting, but can persist for up to 2 weeks. Patients with high degree block that persists beyond this point will require a permanent pacing system. In patients with anterior infarction and high degree block, even if transient, there is a high risk of subsequent asystole and a permanent pacing system implant is recommended.

Late post-infarction arrhythmias

Background

Arrhythmias that develop more than 48 hours after the onset of MI have a different pathophysiology and therapeutic approach. Many of the arrhythmias are related to the formation of fibrosis in the infarct zone. Myocardial fibrosis slows and disturbs conduction, resulting in the development of re-entry circuits that are electrically unstable and generate ventricular tachyarrhythmias. Since these late arrhythmias have a chronic substrate, they are likely to be recurrent. Because of this, they are a common cause of post-infarction mortality, and are a marker of a poor prognosis.

Frequent ventricular ectopic beats

The presence of frequent ventricular ectopic beats in the post-infarction period (>10/h) is strongly associated with an adverse prognosis. More than 100 000 patients have been studied in randomized trials investigating the use of class I and class III antiarrhythmic drugs to suppress ventricular ectopics in the hope of preventing subsequent malignant arrhythmias. None of the large well conducted trials has shown a mortality benefit (and some have shown an adverse pro-arrhythmic effect). In patients with frequent ventricular ectopics, secondary preventative therapy with ACE inhibitors and beta-blockers should be optimized and revascularization performed if there is ongoing ischaemia; antiarrhythmic drug therapy should not be prescribed.

Ventricular tachycardia

Ventricular tachycardia occurring after the first 48 hours, even if asymptomatic or non-sustained, is an important risk factor for early sudden death, particularly when it occurs in association with significant left ventricular dysfunction (ejection fraction <35 per cent). Trials of class I antiarrhythmic drugs have been uniformly disappointing, with no beneficial effect, and some evidence of an adverse pro-arrhythmic effect. In the late 1990s, four important trials (EMIAT, CAMIAT, MADIT and MUST) reported, and provide some guidelines for an evidence-based approach to management of these patients. Based on more than 3000 patients randomized into these trials, we recommend that patients who have ventricular tachycardia after MI (even if asymptomatic or non-sustained) should be considered for autonomic implantable cardioverter defibrillator (AICD) implantation, which will improve their survival. If the patient is not suitable for AICD implantation, then amiodarone is safe and well tolerated for the control of symptomatic arrhythmias (but does not have a proven beneficial effect on mortality).

Thromboembolism and aneurysm formation

Intraventricular thrombi develop in a large proportion of patients with complicated extensive infarcts, often in conjunction with aneurysms. The clinical features associated with an increased risk of thrombosis and aneurysm formation are:

- extensive anterior infarction
- persistent ST elevation in the infarct zone
- heart failure.

Patients with a small MI, particularly if the site is inferior or lateral, are at low risk of these complications. All patients with extensive anterior MI should have an early echocardiogram. If a thrombus is visualized (particularly if it is large, irregularly shaped or has frond-like appendages), there is a substantially increased risk of an early systemic embolus often leading to stroke. Anticoagulation with heparin, followed by warfarin for at least 6 months almost abolishes the risk of a systemic embolism. The risk of systemic embolization declines with time, and warfarin can be withdrawn in selected patients after 6 months. Patients who have an aneurysm associated with heart failure or arrhythmias require early catheterization with a view to CABG and aneurysm resection.

Clinically significant deep venous thrombosis and pulmonary embolism are now rare following uncomplicated MI. The risks are increased in patients with extensive complicated MI, particularly if prolonged bed rest or heart failure occur. In high risk patients, prophylactic low dose subcutaneous heparin (5000 u b.d.) should be instituted and continued until the patient is clinically stable and mobile.

Pericarditis

Pericarditis is an early complication associated with extensive MI, usually within the first week. The clinical features of pericarditis complicating anterior MI are:

- sharp central chest pain, worse with respiration, relieved by sitting up or leaning forward but not relieved by glyceryl trinitrate (GTN);
- an associated friction rub.

In inferior infarction a friction rub is rare, and the pain may be atypical or radiate to the left shoulder. Progression of pericarditis to a clinically significant effusion is rare. Treatment consists of:

- reassuring the patient about the cause of the symptoms;
- pain relief with simple analgesics such as dihydrocodeine, with non-steroidal anti-inflammatory agents reserved for patients with persistent symptoms;
- avoiding administration of anticoagulants if possible, as they may increase the risk of progression to haemorrhagic pericardial effusion, leading to tamponade.

Patients who present later (between 2 weeks and 3 months post-MI) with pericardial pain and friction rub, fever and an elevated erythrocyte sedimentation rate (ESR) may have Dressler's syndrome. This is thought to be an immunological syndrome triggered by myocardial necrosis. Patients may have associated pleurisy and, rarely, pulmonary infiltrates.

Dressler's syndrome is now rare after MI, and is seen most commonly after cardiac surgery.

Recovery and rehabilitation

The in-hospital recovery period

Following admission with MI, all patients should remain on bed rest with continuous rhythm monitoring and close supervision in a CCU environment for at least 24 hours. This is the period of time when the risk of a potentially fatal but reversible arrhythmia is high. In addition, multiple therapeutic interventions designed to reduce infarct size, stabilize the patient and improve prognosis are required. Management after this first 24-hour period will depend on clinical stability and risk profile. Patients who have a small MI (localized ECG changes and small enzyme rise) who are clinically stable with no complications after 24 hours generally have a good prognosis. These uncomplicated patients can begin to mobilize and undertake self-care after 24 hours, and be transferred out of the CCU to a less intensively monitored ward environment. Hospital stay should be limited to around 5 days. By discharge, patients should be walking 200 metres on the level and up a flight of stairs without symptoms. The occurrence of any ischaemia, heart failure, dysrhythmia or other complications during the mobilization phase indicates the need for careful reassessment with a view to determining the need for further investigation prior to discharge.

Patients who have extensive MI (widespread ECG changes and large enzyme rise) are at increased risk of early complications, and remain unstable for a more prolonged period of time. These complicated patients need to stay on CCU for intensive treatment and monitoring, with a large proportion requiring cardiac catheterization, PTCA, cardiac surgery or arrhythmia intervention prior to hospital discharge. High risk patients who are stabilized should be transferred out of CCU with a view to discharge after slow mobilization. Patients and relatives should be provided with verbal and written information about their condition, and referred to a rehabilitation programme.

Risk stratification

Early after MI, risk assessment should be performed to identify patients at increased risk of morbidity and mortality who will benefit from further investigation and treatment. Patients who develop mechanical complications or early recurrent ischaemia usually require investigation and surgical or interventional treatment prior to discharge. In patients who are free of these early complications, increasing age, co-morbidity (particularly diabetes), extensive infarction, and ventricular tachyarrhythmias occurring after the first 48 hours are markers of a poor prognosis. These patients should be considered for early cardiac catheterization or AICD implantation to improve their survival rate. An early echocardiogram can aid risk assessment, helping to identify patients with severe left ventricular impairment [ejection fraction (EF) <35 per cent] and guide prescription of anticoagulant therapy. In patients who survive to hospital discharge, an exercise test should be performed. A symptom-limited Bruce protocol exercise test can be performed on medical therapy 4 weeks after MI. Patients who can complete 9 minutes without chest pain, ischaemic ECG changes or arrhythmias have an excellent prognosis (annual mortality rate around 1 per cent) and do not require further investigation. Patients who fail to achieve a satisfactory workload due to symptoms, easily provocable ischaemia, or arrhythmias should be considered for cardiac catheterization or electrophysiological evaluation to reduce the risk of early adverse events (these patients usually have extensive multivessel disease, and an annual mortality rate of up to 20 per cent which may be reduced by revascularization or arrhythmia control).

Rehabilitation

After MI, cardiac rehabilitation aims to restore patients to their optimal physical, psychosocial, emotional and vocational status using a multidisciplinary and multifactorial programme. Each patient needs a programme tailored to meet individual needs. As a minimum, sessions of medical assessment and review, education and counselling should be offered to all patients. Patients who make a good recovery from their MI and have a satisfactory negative exercise test should enter a supervised exercise programme. In patients with extensive infarction or a positive exercise test, exercise rehabilitation should be deferred until investigation and further treatment are completed. Patients who have important co-morbidity may not be suitable for an exercise programme. Patients who complete a multifactorial rehabilitation programme benefit from:

- reduced anxiety and depression
- increased chance of returning to active employment

- improved cardiovascular function and exercise capacity
- optimized risk factor management.

These beneficial effects combine to improve prognosis, with meta-analysis of over 2000 patients enrolled in randomized studies suggesting that rehabilitation programmes reduce readmission rates and improve mortality by about 25 per cent over 3 years.

Pharmacological secondary prevention

In the absence of contraindications, all patients should receive aspirin and a beta-blocker after MI. Most patients should also receive an ACE inhibitor. Statin therapy has been evaluated in a series of large primary and secondary prevention trials enrolling more than 50 000 patients (CARE, 4S, WOSCOPS, AFCAPS, LIPID and most recently the Heart Protection Study). These trials conclusively demonstrate that:

- statin therapy reduces mortality in patients with symptomatic ischaemic heart disease by around a third;
- statin therapy is safe and well tolerated;
- patients of all ages and either sex benefit;
- patients with relatively normal cholesterol levels obtain similar benefit to those with substantial cholesterol elevation.
- initiation of treatment in hospital helps to reduce the rate of early recurrent ischaemia and readmission.

On the basis of these trial data, all patients with MI should be commenced on a statin during their hospital admission. A starting dose of 40 mg simvastatin (or an equivalent dose of an alternative agent) should be commenced before discharge, with the dose increased during follow-up to reduce cholesterol to less than 4.8 (or by at least 30 per cent in individuals with low starting values). Treatment with aspirin, beta-blockers, and statins should be continued long term.

Lifestyle modification and general advice

Smoking cessation after MI reduces the rate of progression of coronary disease. Cardiac event rates are reduced by 50 per cent. Access to specialized smoking cessation clinics should be available for all smokers. Reducing the number of cigarettes smoked, or changing to cigars or a pipe is not an effective way of reducing risk. Even consumption of one cigarette a day doubles the risk of MI. Passive smoking has a similar adverse effect as smoking one cigarette daily, and partners of MI survivors should be encouraged to stop. A diet low in saturated fat and calories but high in carbohydrates, fruit, vegetables, fibre and fish has favourable effects on lipid profile, blood pressure and haemostatic risk factors, and is recommended after MI. An active lifestyle with regular exercise and stress management techniques improves quality of life and may have beneficial effects on survival. Although consumption of low levels of alcohol may be cardioprotective, high levels of alcohol consumption (more than three units per day) are associated with hypertension and increased mortality, and should be discouraged.

The Driver and Vehicle Licensing Agency (DVLA) does not require that patients inform them after an uncomplicated MI, although patients are not allowed to drive for 4 weeks. After a complicated MI the DVLA may impose a large period of restriction, and patients should be advised to contact the authority directly for advice. The requirements of insurance companies are variable. Patients should seek advice from their own insurer before recommencing driving after MI. Patients who hold a vocational licence to drive an HGV or public service vehicle must contact the DVLA after an MI. These licences will be automatically withdrawn, but may be returned if the DVLA is satisfied with a medical report and the results of a post-MI exercise test (currently patients are required to exercise for 9 minutes of the Bruce protocol, off medical therapy, with no symptoms or ECG changes). Air travel should be avoided for 6 weeks after an uncomplicated MI or longer in patients with complications. Sexual activity should be avoided early after MI. Patients who have a satisfactory exercise test result can be reassured that the cardiovascular demands of intercourse are normally less than of the exercise test, and be encouraged to return to normal activity. Patients with a more complicated MI or significant post-MI exercise symptoms may need more specialized psycho-sexual counselling.

Key points

- MI is very common. Although modern treatment has improved outcome in younger patients, ageing of the population results in a continuing high prevalence of morbidity and mortality.
- Most deaths occur shortly after the onset of symptoms.
- Almost all episodes of MI are caused by thrombotic occlusion of a coronary artery related to an unstable atherosclerotic lesion.
- Plaque instability (reflecting enhanced inflammatory activity within an atherosclerotic lesion) may be triggered by multiple factors.

- Initial diagnosis of acute MI is based on clinical evaluation combined with analysis of the ECG.
- Cardiac troponins are highly sensitive and specific biomarkers, with elevation confirming that irreversible myocardial necrosis has occurred.
- Emergency treatment requires analgesia, oxygen, aspirin, treatment of hypokalaemia and hyperglycaemia and appropriate reperfusion.
- In most units, thrombolysis remains the mainstay of reperfusion therapy, with bolus plasminogen activators (along with adjunctive heparin) offering the best option for achieving rapid easily administered clot lysis.
- Where available, primary PTCA is superior to thrombolysis.
- Beta-blockers, ACE inhibitors and statins should be instituted in all suitable patients.
- Heart failure and hypotension require careful evaluation.
- Mechanical complications are relatively rare but associated with high rates of morbidity and mortality.
- Many arrhythmias are transient and self-terminating. When drug therapy is required, polypharmacy should be avoided.
- Active rehabilitation after MI improves long-term outcome.

Key references

ACE Inhibition Myocardial Infarction Collaborative Group. Indications for ACE inhibitors in the early treatment of acute myocardial infarction. Systemic overview of individual data from 100 000 patients in randomised trials. *Circulation* 1998; **97**: 2202–12.

Anand SS, Yusuf S. Oral anticoagulant therapy in patients with coronary artery disease: a meta-analysis. *JAMA* 1990; **282**: 2058–67.

Brodie BR, Stuckey TD. Mechanical reperfusion therapy for acute myocardial infarction: Stent PAMI, ADMIRAL, CADILLAC and beyond. *Heart* 2002; **87**: 191–2.

Brown N, Young T, Gray D, Skene AM, Hampton JR. Inpatient deaths from acute myocardial infarction, 1982–92: analysis of data in the Nottingham heart attack register. *BMJ* 1997; **315**: 159–64.

Capewell S, Morrison CE, McMurray JJ. Contribution of modern cardiovascular treatment and risk factor changes to the decline in coronary heart disease mortality in Scotland between 1975 and 1994. *Heart* 1999; **81**: 380–6.

Causer JP, Connelly DT. Implantable defibrillators for life threatening ventricular arrhythmias are more effective than antiarrhythmic drugs in selected high risk patients. *BMJ* 1998; **317**: 762–3.

Channer K. Management of the patient after a myocardial infarction. *Prescribers J* 2000; **40**: 20–8.

Channer K, Morris F. ABC of clinical electrocardiography. Myocardial ischaemia. *BMJ* 2002; **324**: 1023–6.

Charles H, Hennekens MD, Christine M *et al.* Adjunctive drug therapy of acute myocardial infarction – evidence from clinical trials. *N Engl J Med* 1996; **28**: 1660–7.

Davey G, Mckeigue P. Insulin infusion in diabetic patients with acute myocardial infarction. *BMJ* 1996; **313**: 639–40.

Davies MJ. The pathophysiology of acute coronary syndromes. *Heart* 2000; **83**: 361–6.

de Belder MA. Acute myocardial infarction: failed thromboysis. *Heart* 2001; **85**: 104–12.

Edhouse J, Brady WJ, Morris F. ABC of clinical electrocardiography. Acute myocardial infarction – Part II. *BMJ* 2002; **324**: 963–6.

Freemantle N, Cleland J, Young P, Mason J, Harrison J. B Blockade after myocardial infarction: systemic review and meta regression analysis. *BMJ* 1999; **318**: 1730–7.

Ghuran A, Camm AJ. Periinfarction arrhythmias. In: Kowey PJ, Podrid PR (eds), *Cardiac Arrhythmias: Mechanisms, Diagnosis and Management.* Philadelphia: Lippincott, Williams and Wilkins, 2001.

Hamm CW, Goldmann BU, Heeschen C, Kreymann G, Berger J, Meinertz T. Emergency room triage of patients with acute chest pain by means of rapid testing for cardiac troponin T or troponin I. *N Engl J Med* 1997; **337**(23): 1648–53.

Hlatky MA. Evaluation of chest pain in the emergency department. *N Engl J Med* 1997; **337**(23): 1687–8.

Mahon NG, O'Rorke C, Codd MB, McCann HA, McGarry K, Sugrue DD. Hospital mortality of acute myocardial infarction in the thrombolytic era. *Heart* 1999; **81**: 478–82.

Malmberg K, Ryden L, Efendic S *et al.* Randomised trial of insulin-glucose infusion followed by subcutaneous insulin treatment in diabetic patients with acute myocardial infarction (DIGAMI study): effects on mortality at 1 year. *J Am Coll Cardiol* 1995; **26**: 57–65.

Morris F, Brady WJ. ABC of clinical electrocardiography. Acute myocardial infarction – Part I. *BMJ* 2002; **324**: 831–4.

Murphy JJ. Problems with temporary cardiac pacing. *BMJ* 2001; **323**: 527.

Nattrass M. Managing diabetes after myocardial infarction. *BMJ* 1997; **314**: 1497.

Noble MIM. Can negative results for protein markers of myocardial damage justify discharge of acute chest pain patients after a few hours in hospital? *Eur Heart J* 1999; **20**: 925–7.

Norris RM. The natural history of acute myocardial infarction. *Heart* 2000; **83**: 726–30.

Ryan TJ, Antman EM, Brooks NH *et al.* 1999 Update: ACC/AHA. Guidelines for the management of patients with acute myocardial infarction: executive summary and recommendations. *Circulation* 1999; **100**: 1016–30.

Tackling myocardial infarction. *Drug Ther Bull* 2000; **38**: 17–22.

The Joint European Society of Cardiology/American College of Cardiology Committee. Myocardial infarction redefined – a consensus document of The Joint European Society of Cardiology/American College of Cardiology Committee for the Redefinition of Myocardial Infarction. *Eur Heart J* 2000; **21**: 1502–13.

The Magnesium in Coronaries (MAGIC) Trial Investigators. Early administration of intravenous magnesium to high risk patients with acute myocardial infarction in the Magnesium in Coronaries (MAGIC) trial. *Lancet* 2002; **360**: 1189–96.

The Task Force on the Management of Acute Myocardial Infarction of the European Society of Cardiology. Acute myocardial infarction: pre-hospital and in-hospital management. *Eur Heart J* 1996; **17**: 43–63.

Topal EJ. Acute myocardial infarction: thrombolysis. *Heart* 2000; **83**: 122–6.

Van der Werf F, Vahanian A, Gulba DC *et al.* Selection of reperfusion therapy for individual patients with evolving myocardial infarction. *Eur Heart J* 1997; **18**: 1371–81.

Wiegers SE, St John Sutton M. When should ACE inhibitors or warfarin be discontinued after myocardial infarction? *Heart* 2000; **84**: 361–2.

Williams SG, Wright DJ, Tan LB. Management of cardiogenic shock complicating acute myocardial infarction: towards evidence based medical practice. *Heart* 2000; **83**: 621–6.

Yusuf S, Anand S, Avezum JR, Flather M, Coutinho M. Treatment for acute myocardial infarction. Overview of randomised clinical trials. *Eur Heart J* 1996; **17**(Suppl F): 16–29.

Zijlstra F. Acute myocardial infarction: primary angioplasty. *Heart* 2001; **85**: 705–9.

Unstable angina

Background

Epidemiology

Unstable angina currently accounts for more than 115 000 acute hospital admissions annually in the UK which is about 200 per 100 000 population. This compares with an estimated 260 myocardial infarction (MI) admissions per 100 000 people. The ratio of male to female patients is about 1.7:1. Prior to 1990, around 20 per cent of patients with unstable angina died or had an MI during their hospital admission. Recent data suggest that the rate of in-hospital death and MI has fallen to less than

10 per cent with modern therapy. One year after the unstable episode, the risk of an adverse event returns to that of a stable patient with a similar risk factor profile.

Definition and classification

The term 'acute coronary syndrome' has been developed to describe the collection of ischaemic conditions which occur through coronary plaque rupture and which includes unstable angina, non-ST segment elevation MI and ST segment elevation MI. The first two patient groups are similar in their mode of presentation and are only distinguished by the finding of raised cardiac enzymes after presentation in the non-ST segment elevation MI group which indicates that the ischaemia caused by the event is severe enough to cause myocardial necrosis.

Unstable angina means that the patient presents with chest pain with the quality of typical angina but these episodes are more severe and prolonged, may occur at rest, or may be precipitated by less exertion than was previously necessary. It is a heterogeneous group of patients, however. The Braunwald classification has been developed to allow the objective description of unstable angina based on the chronological pattern of symptoms, the clinical circumstances and the response to treatment.

- Class I refers to new onset, severe or accelerated angina in patients with angina of less than 2 months' duration which is severe, or which occurs more than three times per day, or is more frequent and precipitated by less exertion. There should be no rest pain.
- Class II describes the presence of angina at rest but is subacute in that patients may have had one or more episodes of angina at rest in the preceding month but not within 48 hours before presentation.
- Class III is angina at rest and is acute with patients having one or more episodes within the last 48 hours.

Patients with recent rest pain (class III) are at increased risk of an early adverse cardiac event.

Pathophysiology

There are several simultaneous processes contributing to the pathophysiology of unstable angina. Angiographic studies have demonstrated complex eccentric morphology consistent with ruptured plaque and superimposed thrombus. Vulnerable plaques that fissure or rupture are characterized by large eccentric lipid pools with foam cell infiltration and tend to rupture at the border of the fibrous cap and adjacent normal intima. This weakness in the integrity of the plaque is initiated by matrix metalloproteinases secreted by macrophages, and ultimately rupture occurs through an acute change in wall shear stress. Intravascular ultrasound studies have confirmed that unstable coronary plaques are associated with more expansive arterial remodelling compared to stable coronary lesions, which may imply a more marked recent progression in extent and severity of plaque at the site of rupture/erosion.

The lipid core is a potent substrate for platelet-rich thrombus formation with the initiation of the coagulation cascade through the interaction of tissue factor with factor VIIa. Platelet adhesion to subendothelial collagen through the release of tissue factor and the expression of the vitronectin ($\alpha_v\beta_3$) receptors leading to platelet activation and aggregation through the expression of the glycoprotein IIb/IIIa receptor is an important event in the development of thrombus. Platelet-rich thrombus is associated with cyclical reductions in coronary blood flow with additional coronary vasoconstriction resulting from endothelial disruption, and thromboxane A_2 (TXA_2) and serotonin production with reduced nitric oxide (NO) production. Inflammatory acute phase proteins, cytokines, and systemic catecholamines stimulate the production of tissue factor, procoagulant activity and platelet hypercoagulability.

There is a strong association between plaque instability and thrombus generation, which contributes to vessel occlusion. However, it is apparent that the thrombus load is less important in an unstable plaque than in a ruptured plaque leading to persistent coronary occlusion, given the lack of benefit with thrombolytic drugs and even the positive harm possible in unstable angina. Recent data have proposed that plaque erosion rather than rupture may explain the difference between an episode of unstable angina and acute MI. Rapid conformational changes in a coronary lesion through proliferation of smooth muscle cells resulting from endothelial injury may occur, decreasing the lumen area, and be exacerbated by erosion of the plaque surface alone.

Risk stratification

The management of unstable angina is different from the acute treatment of ST segment elevation MI. The use of aspirin and a thrombolytic drug has an immediate effect on the acute coronary occlusion associated with MI, but has little effect on subsequent complications such as re-infarction. By contrast, the treatment of unstable angina by medical therapy has limited impact on mortality but leads to a reduction in subsequent infarction or persistent ischaemia. At the time of presentation, it may be difficult to differentiate acute MI from unstable angina. Furthermore, there is a wide heterogeneity of patients presenting with an acute coronary syndrome. The assessment of risk is thus central to the decisions made regarding a conservative or invasive strategy and this should be made on presentation of the patient to the accident and emergency department. Although most patients stabilize with aggressive antianginal therapy, 50–60 per cent of patients still go on to have 'failure' of therapy, either defined as further ischaemia at rest or on early exercise testing.

The characteristics that increase the likelihood of failure of medical therapy are:

- reversible ST segment change
- previous angina
- prior aspirin use
- family history of premature coronary disease
- increased age.

If all these characteristics are present, medical failure occurs in 90 per cent of cases. If none is present, the majority of patients settle with medical therapy.

Clinical features and the 12-lead ECG

The medical history and physical examination provide some help for risk stratification. Patients with multiple risk factors for vascular disease are at increased risk of adverse events. Older age and previous aspirin use are also markers of adverse risk. A highly unstable pattern of symptoms with recent rest pain (Braunwald class III) is also an adverse risk factor. Evidence of haemodynamic instability or compromise indicates a poor prognosis.

The 12-lead electrocardiogram (ECG) is the first key investigation that should be done. The presence of ST segment elevation indicates that the pain is likely to be due to acute MI. Conversely, a completely normal ECG during pain significantly reduces the likelihood that the pain is cardiac in origin. Transient ST segment changes ($\geqslant 0.5$ mm) that develop with symptoms at rest and which resolve with the resolution of symptoms strongly suggests ischaemia. In one study of 773 patients presenting consecutively to hospital within 12 hours of chest pain (without ST segment elevation), 20 per cent had ST segment depression, 26 per cent had inverted T waves, 11 per cent had a non-diagnostic ECG (bundle branch block, paced rhythm) and 43 per cent had a normal initial ECG.

Table 2.1 Short-term risk of death or nonfatal MI in patients with unstable angina

Feature	High risk (at least 1 of the following features must be present)		Intermediate risk (no high risk feature but must have 1 of the following features)	Low risk (no high or intermediate risk feature but may have any of the following features)
History	Accelerating tempo of ischaemic symptoms in preceding 48 hours		Prior MI, peripheral or cerebrovascular disease, or CABG; prior aspirin use	
Character of pain	Prolonged ongoing (>20 minutes) rest pain		Prolonged (>20 minutes) rest angina, now resolved, with moderate or high likelihood of CAD	New-onset CCS class III or IV angina in the past 2 weeks with moderate or high likelihood of CAD
			Rest angina (<20 minutes or relieved with rest or sublingual GTN)	
Clinical findings	Pulmonary oedema, most likely related to ischaemia		Age >70 years	
	New or worsening MR murmur			
	S_3 or new/worsening rales			
	Hypotension, bradycardia, tachycardia			
	Age >75 years			

(Contd)

Table 2.1 (Contd)

Feature	High risk (at least 1 of the following features must be present)	Intermediate risk (no high risk feature but must have 1 of the following features)	Low risk (no high or intermediate risk feature but may have any of the following features)
ECG findings	Angina at rest with transient ST segment changes >0.5 mV	T-wave inversions >0.2 mV	Normal or unchanged ECG during an episode of chest discomfort
	Bundle-branch block, new or presumed new	Pathological Q waves	
	Sustained ventricular tachycardia		
Cardiac markers	Markedly elevated (e.g. TnT or TnI > 0.1 ng/mL)	Slightly elevated (e.g. TnT > 0.01 but < 0.1 ng/mL)	Normal

An estimation of the short-term risks of death and non-fatal cardiac ischaemic events in unstable angina is a complex multivariable problem that cannot be fully specified in a table such as this. Therefore, the table is meant to offer general guidance and illustration rather than rigid algorithms. ACC/AHA Guidelines for the Perioperative Cardiovascular Evaluation for Noncardiac Surgery. *J Am Coll Cardiol* 1996; **27**: 910–48. Reproduced with permission.

Copyright 1996 by the American College of Cardiology and American Heart Association, Inc.

Adapted with permission from Braunwald E, Mark DB, Jones RH et al. *Unstable Angina: Diagnosis and Management*. Rockville, MD: Agency for Health Care Policy and Research and the National Heart, Lung, and Blood Institute, US Public Health Service, US Department of Health and Human Services, 1994. AHCPR Publication No. 94-0602. AHCPR Clinical Practice Guideline No. 10, Unstable Angina: Diagnosis and Management, May 1994.

The PRAIS-UK study was a registry of 1061 patients admitted to 56 hospitals in the UK, half of whom had immediate access to angiography. From this study, the 6-month risk of death or MI was estimated according to age, ECG changes and the presence of heart failure. With age less than 60 years at an odds ratio of 1.0, risk increased to 2.1 for those aged 60–70 and 2.8 for those over 70 years. With a normal ECG having an odds ratio of 1.0, other changes such as T-wave inversion increased the risk to 3.2 and ST segment depression to 5.0, confirming the value of the ECG in determining risk. The presence of heart failure increased risk by 1.9, similar to the twofold risk of being male. In another study, sequential risk for death or MI at 12-month follow-up was evaluated in 911 patients with unstable angina or non-Q wave MI. The risk with a normal ECG, T-wave inversion, ST elevation, ST depression and both ST depression and elevation was 8 per cent, 13 per cent, 15 per cent, 17 per cent and 25 per cent, respectively. The duration of the ischaemia also has a bearing on outcome. Episodes of ischaemia that are associated with ST segment change and persist for 10 minutes or more are associated with the worse prognosis.

Based on these data, a successful algorithm has been developed to triage patients with an acute ischaemic-sounding chest pain. The primary ECG abnormality necessitating admission was ST segment depression or elevation greater than 1 mm. In the presence of lesser changes such as:

- ST elevation 0.5–1 mm
- ST depression 0.25–1 mm
- T-wave inversion in ⩾2 leads
- Q waves
- left ventricular hypertrophy
- abnormal rhythm

a diagnosis of cardiac chest pain was considered likely if the patient was male, pain radiated to neck or left arm, there was nausea/sweating or the patient had a history of previous MI, angina, percutaneous transluminal coronary angioplasty (PTCA) or coronary artery bypass graft (CABG). Where the ECG was normal, three or more of these latter features would be required to increase suspicion of an acute coronary syndrome.

Biochemical markers

Sensitive and specific markers of minor myocardial damage have been identified in recent years, namely the troponin complex. This complex is an integral part of the cardiac myofibril and is released following damage to myocardium. Two regulatory components, troponin I and T, released by myocardial micro-infarction, can be detected peripherally. In MI, troponin levels rise about 4 hours after the onset of chest pain in 30–50 per cent of patients with 100 per cent of infarct patients being positive at 12 hours. A strong relationship exists between the level of peak plasma troponin at 12 hours from the onset of pain and the extent of myocardial damage. Furthermore, several studies have demonstrated that the absolute levels of troponin have a strong relationship to clinical outcome such as death and MI over the short- and medium-term period after presentation with an acute coronary syndrome.

In an early trial in unstable angina, 112 patients with unstable angina were studied: death/MI was 30 per cent in the 39 per cent with an elevated troponin ($>0.2\,\mu g/L$) compared to 2 per cent in the remainder. In the larger Global Utilisation of STreptokinse for Occluded coronary arteries (GUSTO-II) trial, on 865 patients, patients had troponin levels checked. Troponin T elevation predicted adverse outcome particularly death with a relative risk of 17. In a review of 4000 patients with acute ischaemic syndromes, troponin T levels were raised in 33 per cent of patients.

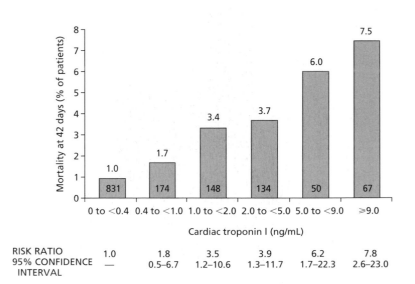

| RISK RATIO | 1.0 | 1.8 | 3.5 | 3.9 | 6.2 | 7.8 |
| 95% CONFIDENCE INTERVAL | — | 0.5–6.7 | 1.2–10.6 | 1.3–11.7 | 1.7–22.3 | 2.6–23.0 |

Figure 2.1 Mortality rates at 42 days according to the level of cardiac Troponin I measured at enrollment. (Reproduced with permission from Antman *et al.*, 1996. Copyright © 1996 Massachusetts Medical Society. All rights reserved.)

The direct relationship between troponin and clinical outcome (mortality) in acute coronary syndromes was shown in a study published in 1996. Mortality at 42 days was 1.0 per cent with a troponin I level <0.4 µg/L compared to 7.5 per cent with a troponin I level ⩾9.0 µg/L (Figure 2.1). In the Fragmin and Fast Revascularization during Instability in Coronary artery disease (FRISC) study, 963 patients participating in a randomized study of low molecular weight heparin (dalteparin) in unstable angina had troponin T measured. A total of 766 patients had a pre-discharge exercise test. Cardiac death or myocardial infarction at 5-month follow-up occurred in 5 per cent, 9 per cent and 13 per cent of patients with a maximum troponin level of 0.06 µg/L, 0.06–0.2 µg/L, and >0.2 µg/L at 12 hours, respectively. Similarly, exercise tolerance and ST segment depression stratified patients into low, intermediate and high risk with death/MI in 5 per cent, 13 per cent and 29 per cent, respectively. Combination of the two variables (troponin T and exercise test) predicted adverse outcome in 1 per cent of low risk, 7 per cent of intermediate risk and 20 per cent of high risk patients (Figure 2.2). Thus, elevation of cardiac troponin indicates

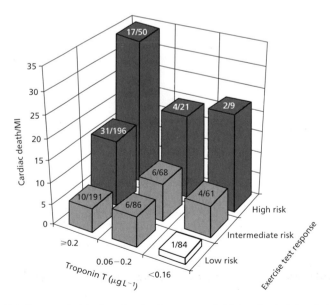

Figure 2.2 Five-month risk of cardiac death or myocardial infarction (MI) in relation to exercise test response and maximal troponin T levels during the first 24 hours. (Reproduced with permission from Lindahl et al., 1997.)

the presence of minor myocyte damage, which is associated with a high risk of subsequent progression to MI and death in patients with unstable angina.

Based on the medical history, physical examination, ECG and biochemical markers, the risk of early major adverse cardiac events such as death, MI or the need for urgent revascularization can be estimated for each individual with unstable angina (Table 2.1, pp. 69–70). Early major adverse events occur in less than 10 per cent of low risk individuals, 10–20 per cent of intermediate risk individuals and 20–40 per cent of high risk individuals. This risk assessment can be further refined using clinical scoring systems such as the TIMI risk score, which assigns points to the presence of different risk factors (with a score of 0–2 indicating low risk, 3–5 intermediate risk and 6–7 high risk). After initial stabilization with drug therapy, patient management is determined by their risk category, as discussed in detail later in this chapter.

Initial management

Immediate management is based on the history, examination, ECG and troponin measurements. The goal from initial assessment of the patient in a monitored environment is to reach a decision regarding the presence or absence of ischaemia, to characterize it as unstable angina or non-ST elevation myocardial infarction and define the next step of discharge, admission or intervention within a period of 6–12 hours.

Patients with definite or possible unstable angina but with a normal ECG and cardiac markers should be observed in a monitored environment where repeat ECG and blood tests can be obtained 12 hours later. If normal, a stress test should be performed either as an in-patient or early after discharge as an out-patient. Low risk patients can be managed as out-patients.

Patients with definite unstable angina and ongoing pain, new ST segment change, new deep T-wave inversion, haemodynamic abnormalities, or a positive stress test should be admitted to a cardiology unit for further management.

Patients with possible unstable angina and negative cardiac markers who cannot exercise or who have resting ECG abnormalities should have a pharmacological stress test.

Patients who develop ST segment elevation should be evaluated for immediate reperfusion therapy.

Drug therapy

The following recommendations should be implemented in the management of patients with an acute coronary syndrome:

- bed rest, with the option for continuous ECG monitoring by telemetry;
- glyceryl trinitrate (GTN), initially sublingual followed by intravenous therapy for the relief of symptoms, if no hypotension present;
- maintenance of adequate oxygen saturation where appropriate;
- opiate analgesia where symptoms are not quickly relieved (by GTN) or where pulmonary oedema supervenes. Care regarding dosing is important in patients with hypotension;
- early beta-blockade in the absence of contraindications (which may be given intravenously if the patient remains in pain followed by oral therapy);
- non-dihydropyridine calcium channel blockade, e.g. verapamil, diltiazem, when beta-blockade is contraindicated;
- aggressive antiplatelet therapy.

In patients with severe continuing ischaemia or frequent ischaemia despite intensive medical therapy or haemodynamic instability, intra-aortic balloon counterpulsation (IABP) may be used before or after coronary angiography.

Nitrate therapy

The main aim of oral and intravenous anti-anginal therapy is to reduce myocardial oxygen demand and improve symptoms of recurrent chest pain. Nitrates are used to reduce chest pain symptoms in unstable patients through a reduction in myocardial oxygen demand (preload and afterload reduction). In addition, nitrates increase coronary collateral blood flow and reduce coronary vasoconstriction. They are of no prognostic benefit. In patients not responding to the use of a sublingual nitrate on three occasions 5 minutes apart, additional benefit from nitrate preparations may be achieved through the initial use of buccal suscard over a period of 20–30 minutes. If this fails to relieve symptoms completely, the patient should receive intravenous nitrate using the regimen detailed in Appendix A. The aim should be to relieve symptoms with a reduction of the mean arterial pressure by 10 per cent. This therapy tends to lose effect after 24 hours through the development of tolerance and it has been suggested that either the dose should be increased or an alternative form of delivery used allowing for a nitrate-free period of 6–8 hours.

Beta-blockers

Beta-blockers diminish the symptoms of ischaemia in patients with stable coronary disease. Although no individual study has demonstrated prognostic benefit in unstable angina, a meta-analysis of 4700 patients receiving beta-blockade confirmed a reduction in MI rate of 13 per cent. The clinical intention of this therapy is to reduce the heart rate to 50–60 b.p.m. If relative contraindications exist, short-acting agents such as metoprolol should be used. It is important to monitor for hypotension and for the development of acute heart failure or bronchospasm.

Calcium channel blockers

Calcium channel blockers can be used to control ischaemia-related symptoms in patients receiving adequate doses of beta-blockade and nitrate, or patients not tolerating both (or either) of these drugs, and in a patients with variant angina. Diltiazem or the dihydropyridine calcium channel blockers (nifedipine, nicardipine) may be added to beta-blockers as additional anti-anginal medication. Because of the tendency to reflex tachycardia through systemic arterial vasodilatation, agents such as nifedipine or nicardipine should not be used as monotherapy (without beta-blockade): a 16 per cent excess in myocardial infarction and recurrent angina has been reported with nifedipine (in the absence of metoprolol). The second-generation dihydropyridines (amlodipine, felodipine) have not been studied in unstable angina. Verapamil and diltiazem have the benefit of inhibiting the sinus (and atrio-ventricular) node, with the former used as an alternative to beta-blockade. It is important to be aware that the combination of beta-blockade and calcium channel blockade can depress left ventricular function.

Aspirin

Aspirin should be administered on presentation with unstable symptoms and continued indefinitely. Aspirin inhibits the cyclooxygenase enzyme in platelets which leads to the formation of thromboxane A2, a potent stimulus to platelet activation. Data from the Veterans Administration

Cooperative Study, the Canadian Multicenter Trial and the Montreal Heart Institute Study confirmed that the use of aspirin in unstable angina reduced the risk of cardiac death and non-fatal MI by 51–72 per cent. From a meta-analysis of seven antiplatelet studies, a 35 per cent reduction in vascular events occurred over 20 months with aspirin. The body of evidence suggests that aspirin should be initiated at a dose of either 160 or 325 mg in patients not already receiving aspirin with subsequent daily dosing at 75–325 mg. With aspirin, however, only one pathway of platelet activation is inhibited and the platelet may also be readily activated by adenosine diphosphate (ADP), thrombin and collagen.

Clopidogrel

In patients who do not tolerate aspirin through hypersensitivity or major gastrointestinal intolerance, a theinopyridine (ticlopidine, or more recently, clopidogrel) should be given. Studies have been undertaken to investigate the role of ticlopidine, which blocks both ADP-mediated platelet aggregation irreversibly and the transformation/ activation of the glycoprotein (Gp) IIb/IIIa receptor which cross-links platelets through fibrinogen. In one study, a 46 per cent reduction in death and non-fatal MI at 6 months (13.6 per cent vs 7.3 per cent, $P < 0.01$) was shown with ticlopidine in addition to conventional therapy. However, its widespread use has been limited by gastrointestinal side effects, a 2.4 per cent risk of neutropenia and 0.8 per cent risk of severe neutropenia.

Clopidogrel, a newer theinopyridine derivative, has the same action as ticlopidine with a more favourable safety profile and evidence for efficacy. A recent major trial, CURE, confirmed the additional value or clopidogrel in the acute coronary syndromes. The trial randomized 12 562 patients with unstable angina/non-ST elevation MI (NSTEMI) to clopidogrel or placebo for 3–12 months (mean of 9 months) in addition to aspirin. Although the trial was done with a conservative ethos, one-third of patients underwent revascularization. Benefit with clopidogrel occurred within the first 24 hours with a 20 per cent reduction in death/MI/cerebrovascular accident (CVA) (primary endpoint), largely driven by a reduction in MI from 6.7 per cent to 5.3 per cent. This was consistent across subgroups and irrespective of revascularization. A relative increase in bleeding risk occurred, 3.7 per cent on clopidogrel compared to 2.7 per cent on placebo. The prospective substudy of patients undergoing percutaneous coronary intervention, PCI-CURE, was reported in 2658 patients. Patients randomized to clopidogrel received it for a mean of 10 days pre-PCI, with both groups receiving open-label clopidogrel for 4 weeks post-PCI usually because of stenting. Prior to PCI, the clopidogrel group had a reduced incidence of MI/refractory ischaemia (12.1 per cent vs 15.3 per cent), which was maintained for the 30 days after PCI – a rate of death/MI/urgent total vascular resistance of 4.5 per cent vs. 6.4 per cent in the placebo pre-treatment group. Of interest, in CURE, the benefit with clopidogrel appeared to occur in addition to the use of GpIIb/IIIa inhibitors. Clopidogrel, like ticlopidine, requires at least 3 days to reach maximum effect but its benefit in the medical management of the acute coronary syndromes is now becoming well established.

Glycoprotein IIb/IIIa receptor antagonists

Because activation of the GpIIb/IIIa receptor is the final common pathway of platelet aggregation through its ability to cross-link with other GpIIb/IIIa receptors through fibrinogen or von Willebrand factor, different agents have been developed specifically to inhibit this process. These are the chimeric (murine–human) antibody fragment to the GpIIb/IIIa receptor, abciximab (Reopro™), synthetic peptides such as eptifibatide (Integrelin™) and synthetic non-peptides such as tirofiban and lamifiban. Abciximab is a F_{ab} antibody fragment of a human–murine (chimeric) monoclonal antibody (c7E3) with a short plasma half-life but with a strong receptor affinity, persisting for weeks (although platelet aggregation returns to normal within 48 hours). Abciximab is relatively non-specific and also inhibits the vitronectin ($\alpha_v\beta_3$) receptor which is on endothelial cells and the MAC-1 receptor on leucocytes. By contrast, the synthetic (small molecule) GpIIb/IIIa receptor antagonists have half-lives of 2–3 hours and are more specific to the receptor.

There is an increased risk of bleeding with these agents, which is typically mucocutaneous or at access sites, particularly at the site of a femoral artery sheath. Based on the experience of the Evaluation of 7E3 for the Prevention of Ischemic Complications (EPIC) trial, the EPILOG trial confirmed the need to reduce the bolus heparin dosing to 70 U/kg during intervention to diminish this risk.

Abciximab

Abciximab has been studied extensively and has clear benefits in patients (stable or unstable) undergoing coronary intervention. The Global Utilization of Streptokinase and t-PA for Occluded Coronary Arteries IV in Acute Coronary Syndromes (GUSTO-IV ACS) trial was designed to investigate whether the use of abciximab has an effect on the clinical outcome of unstable angina independent of coronary intervention. A total of 7800 patients presenting with unstable angina (27–30 per cent with an evolving non-Q-wave MI) were treated with oral aspirin and intravenous heparin or low molecular weight heparin (LMWH) as standard. They were then randomized to either bolus and infusion abciximab or placebo for either 24 or 48 hours. Patients were not scheduled for early coronary intervention unless they became unresponsive to medical therapy. The rate of troponin positivity [troponin T (TnT) >0.1 µg/L] was 58–60 per cent, similar to that seen in the FRISC-II study. This policy resulted in a 48-hour revascularization rate of only 1.6 per cent with this value increasing to 30 per cent after 30 days of follow-up. The primary endpoint of death or MI at 30 days was 8.0 per cent in the placebo group, 8.2 per cent in the 24-hour abciximab group, and 9.1 per cent in the 48-hour abciximab group. Even patients with a raised troponin level or ST segment depression at enrolment showed no benefit with abciximab. There was also an increased need for transfusion in the 48-hour infusion group, 1.3 per cent vs 0.7 per cent ($P < 0.05$).

These data suggest that the benefit of a GpIIb/IIIa receptor drug such as abciximab is only seen if the patient undergoes subsequent intervention largely by reducing the likelihood of peri-procedural MI, rather than being a positive benefit in its own right as a therapy for unstable angina. It has been suggested that the lack of benefit with abciximab compared to the previous interventional studies with the drug may have occurred because the degree of platelet inhibition may have been lower than the target level of >80 per cent over 12 hours, particularly towards the end of the infusion. Alternatively, a prolonged infusion may result in a paradoxical reduction in platelet inhibition.

Tirofiban

Tirofiban is a nonpeptide mimetic of the RGD (arginine-glycine-aspartate) sequence of fibrinogen. In the Platelet Receptor Inhibition in Ischaemic Syndrome Management (PRISM) study, treatment with tirofiban (Aggrastat™) in addition to aspirin and unfractionated heparin reduced death and non-fatal MI at 7 days (4.9 per cent vs 8.3 per cent, $P < 0.01$) and 30 days (8.7 per cent vs 11.9 per cent, $P < 0.01$) but with only a trend at 6 months (12.3 per cent vs 15.3 per cent, $P = 0.06$). Benefit was restricted to those patients who were troponin-positive. In a concurrent trial, PRISM in Patients Limited by Unstable Signs and Symptoms (PRISM-PLUS), 1915 patients with unstable angina/non-ST segment elevation MI received either tirofiban alone, tirofiban with heparin or heparin alone (all with aspirin) for a mean of 71 hours. The tirofiban alone group had an excess of mortality and was discontinued. Angiography was done as clinically indicated. A lower 7-day and 6-month composite endpoint (death/MI/refractory ischaemia) was seen comparing tirofiban and heparin with heparin alone, 12.9 per cent vs 17.9 per cent (32 per cent reduction, $P < 0.01$) and 27.7 per cent vs 32.1 per cent (a 19 per cent reduction, $P < 0.05$), respectively. Extrapolating the 7-day data, which was the primary endpoint, 20 patients would need to receive the combination of drugs to prevent one vascular event at this point. No benefit was seen with tirofiban unless heparin was also given. The benefit of tirofiban and heparin that was present at 7 days on the individual endpoints was lost by 6 months follow-up.

Eptifibatide

Eptifibatide is a cyclic heptapeptide that contains the KGD (lysine-glycine-aspartate) amino acid sequence. In the Platelet glycoprotein IIb/IIIa in Unstable angina: Receptor Suppression Using Integrilin Therapy (PURSUIT) trial, 10948 patients with unstable angina/non-Q-wave MI received heparin, low dose or high dose eptifibatide (Integrilin™) for 72 hours. At 30 days, the composite endpoint of death/non-fatal MI was 14.2 per cent vs 15.7 per cent ($P < 0.05$) in the eptifibatide and placebo group, respectively. This occurred through a non-significant reduction in MI. Taking the patients managed medically without revascularization in North America, the composite endpoint was also reduced with eptifibatide, 14.5 per cent vs 11.8 per cent ($P < 0.05$). The benefit was seen even before PTCA with a reduction in the MI rate, 5.5 per cent vs 1.8 per cent ($P < 0.005$) with placebo and eptifibatide, respectively. Extrapolating the PURSUIT data at 30 days, 67 patients would need to receive both drugs to prevent one vascular event (compared to 31 patients in PRISM-PLUS).

In summary, the early data regarding antiplatelet inhibition with GpIIb/IIIa receptor blockers suggests that the synthetic drugs such as tirofiban and eptifibatide are at their best when given at the outset of presentation of the acute coronary syndrome. By contrast, the data on the benefit during and after percutaneous intervention are much stronger for abciximab than the synthetic drugs. It appears that the benefit of these drugs is restricted to patients with raised troponin levels in an acute coronary syndrome. A trial of the two strategies of either pre-treatment with GpIIb/IIIa receptor antagonists from admission versus administration at the time of intervention is awaited to resolve these contrasting observations.

Antithrombotic therapy

Unfractionated heparin

Placebo-controlled trials of heparin use in unstable angina have been contradictory. In an early landmark study, 479 patients were randomized to received aspirin, heparin, neither, or both over 5 days. A total of 23 per cent of patients on placebo had refractory angina with 12 per cent progressing to MI. In those on heparin alone, only 8.5 per cent had refractory angina while less than 1 per cent had an MI. In another study of 796 patients receiving subcutaneous heparin q.i.d., no improvement in outcome was seen (RISC). A recent meta-analysis of the combination of unfractionated heparin and aspirin for unstable angina suggested a reduction in the risk of MI by 33 per cent, although this initially failed to reach statistical significance until another two studies were added. Until relatively recently, unfractionated heparin was used extensively in acute coronary syndromes but has a variable dose–response curve due to binding to other plasma proteins in addition to antithrombin III. This requires regular monitoring of the activated partial thromboplastin time to maintain a ratio of 1.5–2.5 times control. Furthermore, clot-bound thrombin is unaffected by unfractionated heparin. Unfractionated heparin is also limited by a stimulant effect on platelets and the potential risk of heparin-induced thrombocytopenia.

Low molecular weight heparin

Low molecular weight heparins (LMWH) have a longer plasma half-life with more predictable pharmacokinetics and high bioavailability and can be given subcutaneously. In addition, high ratios of anti-factor Xa to anti-factor IIa lead to potent inhibition of thrombin generation as well as inhibiting thrombin activity. In the Efficacy and Safety of Subcutaneous Enoxaparin in Non-Q-wave Coronary Events (ESSENCE) study, enoxaparin (at a dose of 1 mg/kg b.d.) was shown to be of additional benefit over unfractionated heparin in patients with acute coronary syndromes with an abnormal ECG. The composite endpoint of death/MI/recurrent angina was 19.8 per cent to 16.6 per cent ($P = 0.016$) at 14 days, and 23.3 per cent to 19.8 per cent ($P = 0.016$) at 30 days. No significant difference in death alone was seen. In the ESSENCE trial, enoxaparin was used for a minimum of 3 days and up to 8 days in total. These findings were confirmed in the TIMI IIB study where MI and emergency revascularization were also reduced by enoxaparin, compared to heparin. A meta-analysis of the two trials confirmed a 20 per cent reduction in the rate of death/MI/urgent revascularization and in death/MI at 8, 14 and 43 days. LMWH are associated with more minor bleeding but with no excess in major bleeding risk. The benefit of dalteparin in the FRISC-II study was seen in the group of patients in the early conservative arm, with no significant reduction in events in the early invasive group.

Management after initial stabilization: coronary angiography and exercise testing

In patients with unstable angina, coronary angiography provides anatomical information on the culprit lesion, the extent of disease, global and regional left ventricular function and provides a starting point for subsequent revascularization. On average, angiography will show that:

- 10–20 per cent of patients have no significant epicardial stenosis;
- 30–35 per cent of patients have one vessel disease;
- 5–10 per cent of patients have a significant (> 50 per cent) left main stem stenosis;
- 40–50 per cent have multivessel disease.

There has been debate between proponents for an early invasive strategy compared to an early conservative strategy in the management of unstable angina. An early invasive strategy calls for routine coronary angiography for patients with unstable presenting symptoms without any contraindications to revascularization. An early conservative strategy means that coronary angiography is reserved for patients with evidence of recurrent ischaemia (angina or ST segment changes at rest or on minimal exertion) or a strongly positive exercise tolerance test despite vigorous medical treatment. Early angiography allows risk stratification based on extent of coronary disease and the identification of patients who may benefit prognostically from CABG. Furthermore, coronary intervention will reduce the risk of subsequent hospitalization and the need for multiple anti-anginal drugs compared to a conservative approach. There is a divergence of opinion regarding how early an angiogram is required, however, as some believe that one should proceed to angiography immediately whereas others advocate a period of 12–48 hours of anti-ischaemic and antithrombotic therapy.

High risk patients

The American Heart Association/American College of Cardiology (AHA/ACC) guidelines recommend an invasive strategy in unstable angina in the following situations:

- recurrent angina/ischaemia at rest or low level exercise despite therapy;
- recurrent angina/ischaemia with symptoms or signs of acute heart failure;
- high risk findings on non-invasive stress testing;
- reduced left ventricular function (EF < 40 per cent);
- haemodynamic instability or angina at rest accompanied by hypotension;
- sustained ventricular tachycardia;
- PTCA within the previous 6 months;
- prior CABG;
- patients with repeated presentations with an acute coronary syndrome despite therapy and without ongoing ischaemia or high risk;
- patients older than 65 years of age **or** patients with ST segment depression **or** elevated cardiac markers, with no contraindications to revascularization.

Patients with previous PTCA are likely to have a restenosis best treated with re-intervention and patients with prior CABG represent another subgroup where early angiography may be performed without the need for functional testing. Similarly, patients with reduced left ventricular function, acute heart failure or previous anterior Q-wave MIs have sufficient risk to support a policy of early angiography. Patients with extensive co-morbidities and patients with chest pain with a low likelihood of unstable angina are unlikely to benefit from an invasive strategy.

Intermediate risk patients

Stress testing should take place in this patient group after 2–3 days of freedom from angina. Patients with easily inducible ischaemia require angiography.

Low risk patients

Non-invasive stress testing with a low level treadmill exercise test (two stages of the Bruce protocol) should be performed in patients free of ischaemia at rest or on minimal exertion for 12–24 hours. Should patients be discharged prior to this, symptom-limited exercise testing may be done within 7–10 days of presentation.

Where the baseline ECG has resting ST segment depression ($\geqslant 0.1\,mV$), bundle branch block, left ventricular hypertrophy, an intraventricular conduction defect, a paced rhythm, or the patient is on digoxin therapy, exercise radioisotope perfusion imaging or stress echocardiography may be done to identify a substrate for ischaemia.

Revascularization strategy

PTCA has become an established treatment for unstable angina. The adjunctive use of intracoronary stents and glycoprotein IIb/IIIa receptor antagonists has diminished the risk and improved the outcome associated with PTCA. At present, the rate of in-hospital mortality is still less than 1 per cent with indicators of infarction risk well defined in clinical and angiographic terms.

Historically, in unstable angina coronary artery bypass grafting has been associated with an increased operative mortality at 3.7 per cent (much improved in FRISC-II with an in-hospital mortality of 1.2 per cent) with predictors of risk being left ventricular dysfunction, the need for pre-bypass intra-aortic balloon pumping, and a history of previous CABG. With successful hospital discharge, the 5-year survival is 90 per cent with the greatest relative benefit in those with reduced left ventricular function – in one study in patients with a left ventricular EF <50 per cent, the 3-year mortality was 6.1 per cent in patients after surgery compared to 17.6 per cent in medically treated patients.

The Veterans Affairs Non-Q Wave MI Strategies in Hospital (VAN-QWISH) trial enrolled 920 patients (3 per cent women) with non-Q-wave myocardial infarction and randomized them to either invasive or conservative management. No difference was found in the composite endpoint (death/MI) at 1-year follow-up, 11 per cent invasive group vs 9 per cent conservative group. However, there were some concerns with the true comparison of both arms as only 44 per cent of the invasive group underwent revascularization with mortality especially poor in the remaining 56 per cent. Furthermore, in patients undergoing CABG, there was an excess of major complications (7.7 per cent mortality at 30 days). A total of 64 per cent of patients in the conservative group had an angiogram. These data are also limited by the fact that it occurred in the pre-stent and pre-abciximab era.

The FRISC-II study compared an early invasive and conservative strategy in 2457 patients (3048 eligible) with unstable angina. The patients were of mean age 66 years (70 per cent men). Angiography was performed within 7 days in 96 per cent of the invasive group compared to only 10 per cent of the conservative group. Revascularization (55 per cent PTCA, 45 per cent CABG) was performed within 10 days in 71 per cent of the invasive group compared to 9 per cent of the conservative group, and within 6 months in 77 per cent and 37 per cent, respectively. Comparing the two groups, no difference in Canadian Cardiovascular Society (CCS) angina class was seen with 39 per cent of patients in classes 3–4. There was no difference in troponin T levels (58 per cent $>0.1\,\mu g/L$) with a similar incidence of rest pain, ST segment depression and LMWH use in both groups. There was no excess of clinical adverse events in the invasive group such as groin site bleeding or CVA.

Percutaneous intervention was performed in FRISC-II if one or two flow-limiting lesions were identified. In the invasive group, 522 patients had intervention with a stent rate of 61 per cent and an abciximab usage of 10 per cent. A total of 1.35 ± 0.7 stents were deployed with a primary success rate of 95 per cent at a mean of 4 days (range 2–7) after admission. Demographics were similar in the 220 patients who crossed over from the conservative group other than a mean time to intervention of 16 days (range -132). There was one in-hospital death. Coronary artery bypass surgery was done if three flow-limiting lesions or left main stem disease was identified. Of the 430 patients in the invasive arm, a left internal mammary artery (LIMA) rate of 95 per cent was reported with 85 per cent of patients receiving three or more grafts. There was an in-hospital death rate of 1.2 per cent (compared to 0.4 per cent in the 233 conservative group crossovers) with a 30-day mortality of 2.1 per cent. The mean time to surgery was 7 days (range 5–13) compared to a mean of 28 days in the crossover group.

At 6-month follow-up, the invasive group had a 22 per cent reduction in the composite endpoint of death/MI through a reduction in the rate of MI. Furthermore, there was a reduction in readmission rate by 44 per cent and a 36 per cent reduction in the presence of angina compared to the conservative group. By 12 months, this effect was sustained with a reduction in readmission rate, 37 per cent invasive vs 57 per cent conservative ($P < 0.001$), with a reduced need for further percutaneous intervention, 4.5 per cent invasive vs 16 per cent conservative ($P < 0.001$), or CABG, 3 per cent invasive vs 16 per cent conservative ($P < 0.001$). The primary endpoint of death or MI was reduced by 38 per cent in the invasive group. With respect to angina status, the need for beta-blockade was reduced from 84 per cent to 74 per cent ($P < 0.001$) and the use of oral nitrate from 38 per cent to 17 per cent ($P < 0.001$) in the conservative and invasive groups, respectively. The FRISC-II study also randomized patients to treatment with and without the LMWH dalteparin. The benefit of the adjunctive use of dalteparin was seen in the conservative group with a reduction in primary endpoint, although it had no additional effect on the invasive arm. On subgroup analysis, invasive treatment was of greatest benefit in the elderly, men, those with a longer duration of angina or chest pain at rest and ST segment depression, which is consistent with the recent AHA/ACC guidelines on the management of unstable angina. This improved outcome with an invasive approach was recently confirmed in the TACTICS TIMI 18 and RITA-3 trials.

Antiplatelet therapy as an adjunct to intervention

Abciximab

In addition to intracoronary stenting, the use of specific antiplatelet drugs such as abciximab has improved the outcome in percutaneous intervention in unstable angina, reducing risk from the procedure to the equivalent of elective angioplasty in patients with stable angina. The EPIC trial was an important milestone in the development of novel antiplatelet drugs. A total of 2099 patients enrolled at 56 institutions throughout the USA were scheduled to undergo coronary angioplasty or directional coronary atherectomy and were deemed at risk of abrupt closure on angiographic characteristics, a history of unstable angina with ECG changes within the preceding 24 hours despite medical therapy, or a history of evolving myocardial infarction within the previous 12 hours. All patients were treated with aspirin and heparin and a target activated clotting time (ACT) >300 seconds was achieved during the angioplasty procedure. Patients were assigned to three treatment arms in a randomized fashion:

1 bolus abciximab (0.25 mg/kg) followed by placebo infusion;
2 bolus abciximab (0.25 mg/kg) followed by abciximab infusion (10 μg/kg); and
3 placebo.

The bolus dose was given at least 5 minutes before the procedure and the infusion was continued for 12 hours unless contraindicated. Vascular sheaths were maintained *in situ* for a period of 6 hours after discontinuation of the infusion.

In a subgroup analysis of the main trial, Lincoff *et al.* (1994) documented the particular beneficial effect of abciximab in patients with unstable angina. The 30-day composite primary endpoint (death, myocardial infarction, urgent surgery, or repeat PTCA) was reduced 70.6 per cent by abciximab (bolus plus infusion) in comparison with placebo. The 30-day death rate was 0 vs 3.3 per cent and the myocardial infarction rate was 0.6 vs 9.2 per cent. At 6 months, the death rate was 0.7 vs 6.7 per cent and myocardial infarction rate was 1.3 vs 11.3 per cent. The authors suggested the enhanced benefit of platelet blockade in this group reflects the importance of platelet activity in unstable coronary plaque, which led to the C7E3 Fab Antiplatelet Therapy in Unstable REfractory angina (CAPTURE) trial.

In the CAPTURE trial, 1256 patients with an acute coronary syndrome were randomized to either abciximab or placebo infusion for 18–24 hours prior to and for 1 hour following coronary intervention. The primary endpoint of death/MI/urgent revascularization at 30 days was reduced at 11.3 per cent in the abciximab group compared to 15.9 per cent in the placebo arm ($P = 0.012$). By 6 months, there was no difference in the composite endpoint, however. In this trial, it was noted that the benefit of GpIIb/IIIa inhibition was almost entirely found in patients with a raised troponin level ($>0.1\,\mu g/L$) both before and after intervention. The use of abciximab converted the primary endpoint risk of troponin-positive patients to that of troponin-negative patients (Figure 2.3).

Tirofiban

An early invasive strategy with tirofiban has been reported recently in the Treat angina with Aggrastat and determine Cost of Therapy with an Invasive or Conservative Strategy (TACTICS-TIMI 18) trial (ACC/AHA, 2000). A study population of 2220 patients with an acute coronary syndrome were enrolled from nine countries received aspirin, LMWH, beta-blockade and often statins as well as tirofiban on admission to hospital. They were then randomized either to an invasive strategy with catheterization within 4–48 hours leading to revascularization, or to a conservative group. Tirofiban was administered for 48–108 hours. There was a significant reduction in the primary endpoint of death, MI or re-hospitalization with recurrent unstable angina at 6 months from 19.4 per cent to 15.9 per cent ($P < 0.05$) in the conservative and invasive groups, respectively. This was achieved by a reduction in MI from 6.9 per cent to 4.8 per cent ($P < 0.05$). When analysing the group with positive troponin levels, an absolute reduction in the primary endpoint from 24 per cent to 14 per cent confirmed that a greater benefit from an invasive strategy was seen in higher risk patients.

Eptifibatide

Preliminary data from the Enhanced Suppression of the Platelet Receptor GpIIb/IIIa using Integrilin Therapy (ESPRIT) has been recently reported. Approximately 2400 patients, undergoing PTCA were randomized to receive either placebo or eptifibatide. Eptifibatide was given as two intravenous boluses of $180\,\mu g/kg$ 10 minutes apart

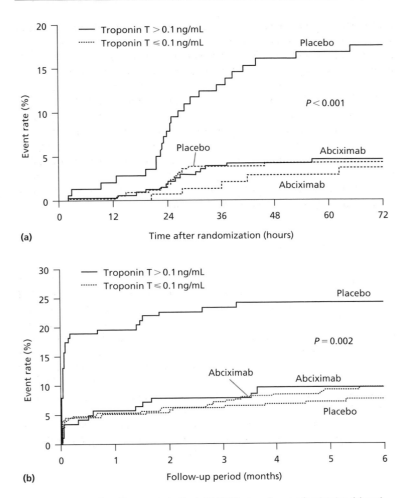

(a)

(b)

Figure 2.3 Rates of cardiac events in the initial 72 hours after randomization (a) and during the 6 months of follow-up (b) among patients with serum troponin T levels above and those with levels below the diagnostic cut-off point. Cardiac events were death and non-fatal infarction. Percutaneous transluminal coronary angioplasty was performed 18–24 hours after randomization. (Reproduced with permission from Hamm *et al.*, 1999. Copyright © 1999 Massachusetts Medical Society. All rights reserved.)

with a $2\,\mu g/kg/min$ infusion maintained for up to 24 hours (a higher dose than given in PURSUIT). In patients within 7 days of a ST segment elevation MI, and in patients with an acute coronary syndrome for less than and more than 2 days, the relative reduction in the risk of death/MI/urgent revascularization was 44 per cent, 47 per cent, and 48 per cent, respectively. This compares with a relative reduction of 25 per cent in patients with stable angina. The benefit was greatest in patients with a raised troponin level: the incidence of a major adverse cardiac event (MACE) at 48 hours and 30 days was 12.2 per cent vs 4.2 per cent and 13.5 per cent vs 5.6 per cent in the placebo and eptifibatide groups, respectively. Greater benefit was also seen in patients with a raised CK-MB fraction implying recent non-Q-wave myocardial infarction.

There is a large body of evidence to support the use of GpIIb/IIIa inhibitors as an adjunctive therapy in unstable patients undergoing intervention. Recently published guidelines by the National Institute of Clinical Excellence (NICE) support their use in troponin-positive patients undergoing coronary intervention.

Post-discharge care

It is important that patients who have been admitted with an acute coronary syndrome should have follow-up determined by their initial risk and mode of therapy. Low risk patients treated medically and revascularized patients should be reviewed within 6 weeks and higher risk patients should be seen sooner within a 2-week period of discharge. If patients treated conservatively develop more unstable symptoms or significant stable symptoms on exercise less than 400 metres (CCS class III) angina, they should be considered for revascularization. In addition, patients with clinical or echocardiographic evidence of left ventricular dysfunction should receive an ACE inhibitor.

All appropriate risk factors such as LDL-cholesterol level, hypertension, hyperglycaemia in diabetics, weight and smoking habit should be modified according to accepted guidelines.

Considerations in special groups

Diabetes mellitus

Diabetes is an independent risk factor for coronary heart disease events and this should be taken into account in the initial risk stratification of the patient. Diabetics have more extensive disease, more unstable lesions, other co-morbidities, and less favourable results from revascularization, especially PTCA. Data from the EPISTENT study confirmed that should these patients undergo PTCA, significant mortality benefit occurred with the adjunctive use of abciximab.

Post-CABG patients

These patients account for 20 per cent of unstable patients and are at higher risk given more extensive disease and left ventricular dysfunction. Saphenous vein graft degeneration increases with time and indicates the highest risk substrate for PTCA where grafts are older than 5 years.

Elderly patients

This group has more atypical modes of presentation, more co-morbidities, less definitive ECG stress tests and differential responses to drug therapy. Outcomes from revascularization are less good than in younger patients and PTCA may be a reasonable strategy even in diffuse disease given the lower morbidity from this procedure. The general medical status of the patient as well as anticipated life expectancy should be taken into account when planning a treatment strategy.

Variant angina

This is a specific form of unstable angina characterized by transient ST segment elevation caused by focal coronary artery spasm at the site of significant endothelial dysfunction and hypersensitivity. It is important to differentiate this clinical presentation from the early stages of acute MI from plaque rupture, which is far commoner. Coronary spasm responds to sublingual nitrates, long-acting nitrates and calcium channel blockade, and the latter should be given at high doses, e.g. verapamil 480 mg/day, diltiazem 360 mg/day, nifedipine 120 mg/day, as maintenance therapy. Coronary arteriography is indicated in patients with episodic chest pain and ST segment elevation. In such patients, where no obstructive lesion is demonstrated, provocative testing, e.g. with ergonovine or acetylcholine, is appropriate.

New developments

Statin therapy

The benefit of statin therapy in the primary prevention of coronary heart disease and in the secondary prevention of further events in patients with angina, and previous unstable angina or infarction is well established. There is some evidence to support their role as adjunctive therapy in acute coronary syndromes. The rationale for this is based on their pleiotropic effects such as a positive effect on endothelial function, a reduction in platelet aggregability and an anti-inflammatory effect, manifest as a reduction in the C-reactive protein level. In the RECIFE study, 60 patients were randomized to pravastatin 40 mg or placebo at a mean of 10 days following MI or unstable angina. Flow-mediated dilatation increased by 42 per cent in the pravastatin group after 6 weeks of treatment. In the L-CAD study, 126 patients with post-MI angina underwent coronary angioplasty and then were randomized to 20–40 mg pravastatin or placebo. At 2 years, there was a reduction in death/MI/revascularization, 27 per cent vs 52 per cent ($P < 0.05$) in the statin-treated and placebo group, respectively.

Most recently, the Myocardial Ischaemia Reduction with Aggressive Cholesterol Lowering (MIRACL) trial reported 3000 patients with an acute coronary syndrome (excluding ST segment elevation MI) who were randomized to either atorvastatin 80 mg or placebo within 63 hours of presentation, in addition to routine anti-ischaemic therapy. At 4-month follow-up, there was a reduction in the composite endpoint of death/MI/resuscitated cardiac arrest/re-hospitalization for worsening angina from 17.4 per cent to 14.8 per cent ($P = 0.048$). As a secondary endpoint, the latter variable was the one outcome reduced by this therapy. Based on the evidence for statin therapy in acute coronary syndromes, the Pravastatin or Atorvastatin Evaluatin and Infection Therapy (PROVE-IT) study has been designed to compare pravastatin 40 mg with atorvastatin 80 mg (both with and without antibiotics) in patients within 10 days of an acute coronary syndrome with follow-up over 18 months.

Key points

- An acute coronary syndrome is a collective term that describes the ischaemic conditions which occur through acute coronary plaque rupture or erosion, which includes unstable angina and non-ST segment elevation myocardial infarction, and is often expanded to include ST segment elevation myocardial infarction.
- Around 10 per cent of patients with unstable angina will have an in-hospital major adverse cardiac event (death, MI, or refractory ischaemia). In the next 6 months, a further 25 per cent will have a major adverse event.

- Unstable angina patients comprise a heterogeneous group presenting with new onset, worsening or rest angina and can be classified according to chronological pattern of symptoms, clinical presentation and response to treatment.
- Patients with unstable angina can be risk-stratified according to presenting variables such as age, presence of cardiovascular risk factors, presence of coronary disease, ECG appearance, clinical history, pre-existing drug therapy and the elevation of biochemical markers of myocardial injury.
- Initial medical assessment of an unstable patient includes an accurate history and examination, 12-lead ECG and measurement of cardiac troponin level.
- Initial treatment involves bed rest, nitrate, low molecular weight heparin beta-blocker and antiplatelet therapy.
- The ESSENCE trial confirmed the clinical benefit of low molecular weight heparin (enoxaparin for 3–8 days) over unfractionated heparin with a reduction in the composite endpoint of death/MI/recurrent angina at 30 days. The CURE trial confirmed the additional value of the antiplatelet drug, clopidogrel, in the management of acute coronary syndromes that appeared to occur in addition to the use of GpIIb/IIIa inhibitors.
- The benefit of the GpIIb/IIIA receptor inhibitor abciximab is greatest in patients with an acute coronary syndrome undergoing subsequent percutaneous coronary intervention where a mortality benefit has been demonstrated over long-term follow-up. The small molecule GpIIb/IIIa receptor inhibitors, eptifibatide and tirofiban, are also of clinical benefit in unstable patients, but again, particularly in those undergoing intervention.
- Patients with high or intermediate risk should be considered for coronary angiography and early revascularization and this will lead to a reduction in subsequent myocardial infarction, recurrent ischaemia and hospitalization.

Key references

ACC/AHA guidelines for the management of patients with unstable angina and non-ST segment elevation myocardial infarction: executive summary and recommendations. *Circulation* 2000; **102**: 1193–209.

Ambrose JA, Winters SL, Stern A *et al*. Angiographic morphology and the pathogenesis of unstable angina pectoris. *J Am Coll Cardiol* 1985; **5**: 609–16.

Anderson HV, Cannon CP, Stone PH et al. One year results of the Thrombolysis in Myocardial Infarction (TIMI) IIIB clinical trial. J Am Coll Cardiol 1995; 26: 1643–50.

Antiplatelet Trialists Collaboration. Collaborative overview of randomised trials of antiplatelet therapy – 1: Prevention of death, myocardial infarction, and stroke by prolonged antiplatelet therapy in various categories of patients. BMJ 1994; 308: 81–106.

Antman EM, Cohen M, Bernink PJ et al. The TIMI risk score for unstable angina/non-ST elevation MI: a method for prognostication and therapeutic decision making. JAMA 2000; 284: 835–42.

Antman EM, Tanasijevic MJ, Thompson B et al. Cardiac-specific troponin I levels to predict the risk of mortality in patients with acute coronary syndromes. N Engl J Med 1996; 335: 1342–9.

Armstrong PW, Fu Y, Chang W-C et al. Acute coronary syndromes in the GUSTO IIb trial: prognostic insights and impact of recurrent ischemia. Circulation 1998; 98: 1860–8.

Boden WE, O'Rourke RA, Crawaford MH et al. Outcomes in patients with acute non-Q wave myocardial infarction randomly assigned to an invasive as compared with a conservative management strategy. N Engl J Med 1998; 338: 1785–92.

Cohen M, Demers C, Gurfinkel EP et al. A comparison of low molecular weight heparin with unfractionated heparin for unstable coronary artery disease. N Engl J Med 1997; 337: 447–52.

The Danish Study Group on Verapamil in Myocardial Infarction. Effect of verapamil on mortality and major events after acute myocardial infarction (the DAnish Verapamil Infarction Trial II – DAVIT II). Am J Cardiol 1990; 66: 779–85.

Hamm CW, Heeschen C, Goldmann B et al. Benefit of abciximab in patients with refractory unstable angina in relation to serum troponin T levels. N Engl J Med 1999; 340: 1623–9.

Hamm CW, Ravkilde J, Gerhardt W et al. The prognostic value of serum troponin T in unstable angina. N Engl J Med 1992; 327: 146–50.

Invasive compared with non-invasive treatment in unstable coronary-artery disease: FRISC II prospective randomised multicentre study. FRagmin and Fast Revascularisation during InStability in Coronary artery disease Investigators. Lancet 1999; 354: 708–15.

Lincoff AM, Califf RM, Anderson K, Weisman HF, Topol EJ, for EPIC Investigators. Striking clinical benefit with platelet GP IIb/IIIa inhibition by c7E3 among patients with unstable angina: outcome in the EPIC trial. Circulation 1994; 90: I-21.

Lindahl B, Andrén B, Ohlsson J, Venge P, Wallentin L and the FRISK study group. Risk stratification in unstable coronary artery disease: additive value of troponin T determinations and pre-disharge exercise tests. Eur Heart J 1997; 18: 762–70.

Mehta SR, Yusuf S, Peters RJG et al. Effects of pretreatment with clopidogrel and aspirin followed by long-term therapy in patients undergoing percutaneous coronary intervention: the PCI-CURE study. Lancet 2001; 358: 527–33.

Oler A, Whooley MA, Oler J et al. Adding heparin to aspirin reduces the incidence of myocardial infarction and death in patients with unstable angina. A meta-analysis. *JAMA* 1996; **276**: 811–15.

O'Shea JC, Buller CE, Cantor WJ et al., for the ESPRIT Investigators. Long-term efficacy of platelet glycoprotein IIb/IIIa integrin blockade with eptifibatide in coronary stent intervention. *JAMA* 2002; **287**: 618–21.

Randomised placebo-controlled trial of abciximab before and during coronary intervention in refractory unstable angina: the CAPTURE Study. *Lancet* 1997; **349**: 1429–35.

Rottbauer W, Greten T, Müller-Bardorff M et al. Troponin T: a diagnostic marker for myocardial infarction and minor cardiac cell damage. *Eur Heart J* 1996; **17**(Suppl F): 3–8.

Stone PH, Thompson B, Zaret BL et al. Factors associated with failure of medical therapy in patients with unstable angina and non-Q wave myocardial infarction: a TIMI-IIIB database study. *Eur Heart J* 1999; **20**: 1084–93.

The CURE investigators. Effects of clopidogrel in addition to aspirin in patients with acute coronary syndromes without ST segment elevation. *N Engl J Med* 2001; **345**: 494–502.

The EPIC Investigators. Use of a monoclonal antibody directed against the platelet glycoprotein IIb/IIIa receptor in high risk coronary angioplasty. *N Engl J Med* 1994; **330**: 956–61.

The EPILOG Investigators. Platelet glycoprotein IIb/IIIa receptor blockade and low-dose heparin during percutaneous coronary revascularization. *N Engl J Med* 1997; **336**: 1689–96.

The RISC group. Risk of myocardial infarction and death during treatment with low dose aspirin and intravenous heparin in men with unstable coronary artery disease. *Lancet* 1990; **336**: 827–30.

Theroux P, Ouimet H, McCans J et al. Aspirin, heparin or both to treat acute unstable angina. *N Engl J Med* 1988; **319**: 1105–11.

Théroux P, Taeymans Y, Morissette D, Bosch X, Pelletier GB, Waters DD. A randomized study comparing propranolol and diltiazem in the treatment of unstable angina. *J Am Coll Cardiol* 1985; **5**: 717–22.

Topol EJ, Califf RM, Weisman HF et al., for the EPIC investigators. Randomised trial of coronary intervention with antibody against platelet IIb/IIIa integrin for reduction of clinical restenosis: results at six months. *Lancet* 1994; **343**: 881–6.

Wallentin L, Lagerqvist B, Husted S et al. Outcome at 1 year after an invasive compared with a non-invasive strategy in unstable coronary-artery disease: the FRISC II invasive randomised trial. FRISC II Investigators. Fast Revascularisation during Instability in Coronary artery disease. *Lancet* 2000; **356**: 9–16.

Yusuf S, Wittes J, Friedman L. Overview of results of randomized clinical trials in heart disease. II. Unstable angina, heart failure, primary prevention with aspirin, and risk factor modification. *JAMA* 1988; **260**: 2259–63.

Resuscitation

3

Background

Epidemiology and physiology

Cardiovascular disease is the leading cause of death in the UK, with more than 300 000 victims each year. Sudden cardiac death represents approximately 25–30 per cent of all cardiovascular death, claiming an estimated 70 000–90 000 lives each year.

Although the causes of cardiac arrest are numerous (Box 3.1), most events in adults occur as a result of ischaemic cardiovascular disease. A number of studies have shown a circadian pattern of cardiac arrest with the majority of events occurring in the morning hours (6 a.m. to 12 noon) and a low incidence at night. Some data also suggest a late afternoon peak between 4 p.m. and 7 p.m. A seasonal variation in cardiac arrest is also recognized with an increased number of cases occurring during the winter months. Resuscitation after cardiopulmonary arrest is effective in only one in five patients with about a third of long-term survivors having apparent motor or cognitive deficits.

By far, the most commonly encountered rhythm is ventricular fibrillation (VF) or pulseless ventricular tachycardia (VT) occurring in more

Box 3.1 Some causes of VF/pulseless VT, asystole and pulseless electrical activity (PEA)

Ventricular fibrillation
Reversible triggers
Acute myocardial infarction/ischaemia
Electrolyte disturbances (hypokalaemia, hyperkalaemia, hypocalcaemia, hypomagnesemia, metabolic acidosis, etc.)
Drugs (antiarrhythmics, phenothiazines, tricyclic antidepressants, digoxin toxicity, etc.)
Illicit drug use, e.g. cocaine, amphetamines, ecstasy (see Chapter 9)
Commotio Cordis (see Chapter 11, cardiac trauma)
Electric shock

Structural heart disease
Coronary artery disease
- Atherosclerotic
- Non-atherosclerotic (Prinzmetal angina, anomalous origin of coronary artery, etc.)

Cardiomyopathies
Valvular heart disease
Myocarditis
Congenital heart disease
Arrhythmogenic right ventricular dysplasia
Primary pulmonary hypertension
Infiltrative heart disease (amyloidosis, sarcoidosis, tumour)

Structurally normal heart
Wolff–Parkinson–White syndrome
Long QT syndromes
Brugada syndrome
Idiopathic VT/VF

Asystole
Heart block
Myocardial infarction
Hypoxia
Drugs (antiarrhythmics, beta-blockers, verapamil) especially with pre-existing sinus node disease

Pulseless electrical activity (PEA)
'4 Hs and 4 Ts'
Hypoxia
Hypovolaemia
Hypo/hyperkalaemia and other metabolic disorders
Hypothermia
Tension pneumothorax
Tamponade
Toxic/therapeutic disorders
Thromboembolic and mechanical obstruction

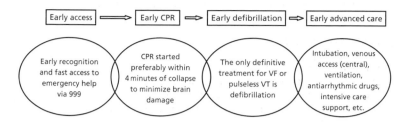

Figure 3.1 The key to a successful resuscitation outcome is dependent on a rapid sequence of events with minimal delay.

than 50 per cent of cases. With time, VF deteriorates from coarse VF to fine VF and eventually to asystole. The prognosis is less favourable for non-VF/VT rhythms. Independent predictors of mortality during follow-up include increased age ($\geqslant$65 years), the presence of heart failure and cardiac arrest not due to a definite myocardial infarction (MI).

After a cardiac arrest, the only interventions that have been proven to improve long-term survival are basic life support and early defibrillation [immediate commencement of cardiopulmonary resuscitation (CPR) confers a 2.7-fold increase in the rate of survival]. Therefore, the key to a successful outcome is dependent on initiation of a rapid sequence of events with minimal delay (Figure 3.1). Ideally, the goal of in-hospital defibrillation should be a collapse–shock interval of less than 3 minutes. Although data from randomized controlled trials are limited, techniques for CPR have been standardized in recent years, and the guidelines in this chapter are based on those published by the Resuscitation Council (UK) and the European Resuscitation Council (ERC).

The major role of CPR is to provide some blood flow to both the myocardium and central nervous system to allow for successful defibrillation and resuscitation, and to preserve long-term organ function. Although a number of theories have been proposed, the mechanism by which external chest compression provides an artificial circulation is not fully known. Even when performed optimally, chest compression does not achieve more than 30 per cent of the normal cardiac output. One of the most important concepts in understanding the physiology of CPR is that of coronary perfusion pressure. Coronary perfusion pressure is defined as the difference between the aortic diastolic pressure and the right atrial pressure (the venous return of myocardial flow is through the great cardiac vein, coronary sinus and eventually the right atrium, therefore an increase in right atrial pressure may impede venous run-off from the myocardial capillary bed). The majority of coronary flow occurs during artificial diastole or the chest relaxation phase of

CPR, and is dependent on the coronary perfusion pressure. Experimental studies have shown that the larger the coronary perfusion pressure, the greater the coronary blood flow, and the greater the chance for a successful outcome. The coronary perfusion pressure can be optimized by increasing the peripheral vascular tone using vasoconstrictors such as adrenaline, or by increasing the number of chest compressions per minute. A compression rate of 100 per minute is currently recommended by the ERC, partly due to concerns that higher rates may be physically too exhausting for members of the arrest team.

During cardiac arrest and CPR, a severe mixed acidosis can develop. A reduction in alveolar gaseous exchange because of an increase in dead space and a decrease in lung compliance (due to pulmonary oedema) can lead to respiratory acidosis. The combination of circulatory collapse and poor tissue perfusion can result in marked metabolic acidosis. Severe acidosis is negatively inotropic, causes electrolyte disturbances and can cause intractable arrhythmias and a poor resuscitation outcome.

The ABC of resuscitation and specific interventions

The ABC of resuscitation begins with basic life support and the establishment of an adequate airway (A), breathing (B) and circulation (C). The purpose of basic life support is to maintain adequate ventilation and circulation until advanced techniques can be applied to reverse the underlying cause of the arrest. It is assumed that a sound knowledge in basic life support already exists, and therefore this chapter concentrates mainly on management issues and interventions during advanced life support.

Airway

A quick inspection of the oropharynx should be performed, and any obstructions such as food or loose dentures should be removed. Tight-fitting dentures should be left as it helps support the soft palate. Manoeuvres such as the head tilt, chin lift and jaw thrust can be used to ensure that the tongue and soft tissues do not obstruct the airway. A variety of airway adjuncts are now available on most resuscitation trolleys and include facial masks, Guedel airways (an estimate of the size may be obtained by selecting an airway with a length corresponding to the distance between the corner of the patient's mouth and the angle of the jaw) and nasopharyngeal tubes (the diameter size in adults is usually 6–7 mm or the diameter of the little finger). The tip of a nasopharyngeal tube should be visible in the pharynx behind the tongue. For more skilled and experienced staff, the insertion of a laryngeal mask or, ideally, an endotracheal tube can be attempted.

Breathing

It is important to look, listen and feel for breath sounds and chest movements. In any patient in whom breathing is inadequate or absent, artificial ventilation must be commenced as soon as possible. Oxygenation of the patient is the primary objective and the highest concentration of oxygen available should be administered. This can be achieved by using a mask with a reservoir bag, which can deliver inspired oxygen concentrations of 85 per cent at flow rates of 10–15 L/min. Tidal volumes of 400–600 mL are adequate to make the chest rise and are less likely to cause gastric insufflation and aspiration. Between 1.5 and 2 seconds should be spent in the inspiratory phase.

Circulation

Until now, previous resuscitation guidelines have required the absence of a carotid pulse to diagnose cardiac arrest and start CPR. However, times in excess of 30 seconds are required to achieve an accuracy of 95 per cent. As a consequence, current guidelines have de-emphasized the carotid pulse as the sole criterion for starting CPR, and include the search for signs of a circulation such as any movement, including swallowing and breathing. If there is no circulation, then chest compressions should be commenced by first locating the xiphisternum, with the middle finger, then placing the index finger of the same hand on the sternum superior to the middle finger. The heel of the other hand slides down the sternum until it reaches the index finger. The heel of one hand is placed in this position, with the other hand on top of the first. The fingers should be off the chest and interlocked. Vertical downward pressure is applied to depress the sternum 4–5 cm and then the pressure is released. A compression rate of 100 per minute using a compression to ventilation ratio of 15:2 is now recommended for single and multiple rescuers when ventilating non-invasively (bag and mask). Once intubated, ventilation should continue at approximately 12 breaths/ min and chest compression maintained uninterrupted for ventilation. Uninterrupted chest compression results in substantially higher mean coronary perfusion pressure.

Defibrillation

The only definitive treatment for VF or pulseless VT is defibrillation. Although these rhythms are initially readily treatable, the chances of successful defibrillation diminish rapidly with time and decline by 7–10 per cent per minute. Therefore, the priority is to minimize any delay between the onset of cardiac arrest and the administration of defibrillation shocks. For witnessed arrests, especially in patients with cardiac monitoring, a precordial thump to the patient's sternum can be given. The thump delivers a small amount of kinetic energy, which may be adequate to convert a fibrillating myocardium. VF or pulseless VT greater than 30 seconds is unlikely to respond to a precordial thump and electrical cardioversion is required. Shocks are initially started at 200 J, as this energy level is capable of defibrillation with minimal damage to the heart. The first shock lowers transthoracic impedance, allowing the second 200 J shock to be more effective. If these shocks are unsuccessful, then higher energy shocks of 360 J are given. Shocks greater than 360 J are likely to cause myocardial injury. The paddles should be left on the patient's chest while the defibrillator is recharged, at the same time observing the electrocardiogram (ECG) monitor for any change in the rhythm. During resuscitation, if defibrillation results in a change of rhythm that restores circulation, and later reverts back to VF or pulseless VT, then the algorithm is reapplied from the beginning, i.e. 200 J. Successful defibrillation is dependent on maximizing the current flow that traverses the myocardium. This can be achieved by ensuring correct paddle positions (Figure 3.2a) with firm pressure being applied to the chest wall, application of proper coupling agents to aid the passage of current at the interface between the paddle and chest wall, and defibrillating during the expiratory phase of ventilation. If defibrillation is unsuccessful in the anterolateral position, then further attempts in the anteroposterior position (Figure 3.2b) and/or a different defibrillator are worth trying. The positions of the positive and negative paddles do not matter when defibrillating.

In patients with permanent pacemakers, defibrillation in the anteroposterior position is preferable. Although modern pacemakers are fitted with protection circuits, if anterolateral defibrillation is attempted, ensure that the electrodes are placed at least 12–15 cm from the pacemaker unit.

Pacing

Pacing can often be life saving, especially in situations where bradycardia preceded the cardiac arrest or where bradycardia is associated with

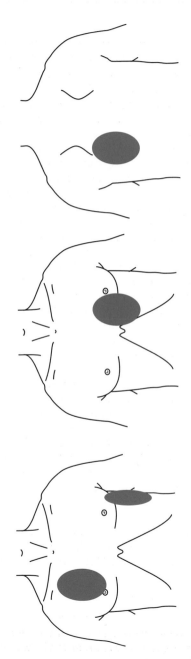

Anterior-lateral electrode position for defibrillation and/or transcutaneous cardiac pacing

One electrode is placed to the right of the upper sternum below the clavicle.
The other electrode is placed at the level of the fifth intercostal space in the anterior axillary line (corresponding to V5–V6 ECG electrode).

(a)

Anterior-posterior electrode position for defibrillation and/or transcutaneous cardiac pacing

One electrode is placed to the left of the lower sternal border (corresponding to V2 and V3 ECG electrode). The other electrode is placed beneath the scapula, lateral to the spine on the left, at the same level as the anterior electrode.

(b)

Figure 3.2 Paddle positions for anterior-lateral and anterior-posterior defibrillation.

haemodynamic intolerance following successful resuscitation. Pacing can be attempted non-invasively or invasively, depending on the equipment available and/or the experience of the operator.

NON-INVASIVE (TRANSCUTANEOUS) PACING

Transcutaneous pacing can be easily applied, requires minimum training and avoids the risks of central venous cannulation. Many defibrillators are now equipped with external pacing facilities and it is important for those involved in managing cardiac arrest to familiarize themselves with this option. In short, any excess chest hair should be removed by clipping. Shaving the chest may cause tiny nicks in the skin, which may increase patient discomfort during pacing. If the transcutaneous pacing system is limited to pacing alone, then the anterior-posterior electrode configuration is used (placing the negative electrode anteriorly and the positive electrode posteriorly) (Figure 3.2b). Hence, if defibrillation is required it can easily be done in an anterolateral position, without interfering with the pacing electrode. If the life pack is a modern multifunction defibrillator-pacemaker then the anterolateral configuration (positive electrode at the right upper sternum and the negative electrode in the anterior axillary line) can be used (Figure 3.2a). The ECG gain is adjusted to ensure sensing of any intrinsic QRS complexes. The demand mode is selected and the pacing rate set to 60–90 b.p.m. The pacing current is set at the lowest setting and the pacemaker turned on. The current is then slowly increased, observing the patient, and monitored until electrical capture is seen. As the current increases, the skeletal muscles contract and a pacing spike is seen on the monitor. Electrical capture is recognized by wide QRS complex and a broad T wave and a current range of 50–100 mA is usually sufficient (Figure 3.3). The presence of a palpable pulse ensures electrical capture results in mechanical capture (myocardial contraction). Failure to achieve mechanical capture in the presence of good electrical capture indicates non-functional myocardium. Patients often require sedation with an IV benzodiazepine (Diazemuls) as the procedure can be painful. Transcutaneous pacing is only a temporary measure until transvenous pacing can be instituted.

TRANSVENOUS PACING (BOX 3.2)

The resuscitation trolley should always be present and venous access available. Bradycardia, asystole and ventricular tachyarrhythmias are often induced during the procedure, and therefore atropine, isoprenaline and lignocaine should be readily at hand. The commonest route for placing a temporary wire is usually the right subclavian vein (the left side is then available for a permanent implant if required). The risk

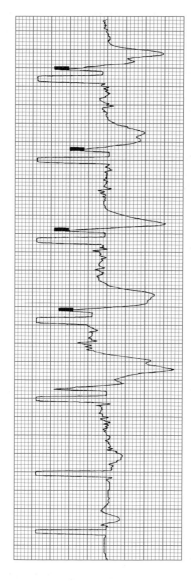

Figure 3.3 Non-invasive transcutaneous pacing. The first two pacing spikes are not followed by a QRST wave complex and therefore signify failure to capture. The remaining pacing spikes demonstrate ventricular capture. It is important to ensure that electrical capture is associated with mechanical capture by the presence of a palpable pulse.

Box 3.2 Indications for temporary transvenous cardiac pacing

Emergency/acute

Acute myocardial infarction
- Asystole
- Symptomatic bradycardia (sinus bradycardia with hypotension and Mobitz type I second degree AV block with hypotension not responsive to atropine)
- Bilateral bundle branch block (alternating BBB or RBBB with alternating LAHB/LPHB)
- New or indeterminate age bifascicular block with first degree AV block (trifascicular block)
- Mobitz type II second degree AV block
- Overdrive suppression of tachyarrhythmias

Bradycardia not associated with acute myocardial infarction
- Asystole
- Second or third degree AV block with haemodynamic compromise or syncope at rest
- Ventricular tachyarrhythmias secondary to bradycardia

Elective
- Support for procedures that may promote bradycardia
- General anaesthesia with:
  – second or third degree AV block
  – intermittent AV block
  – first degree AV block with bifascicular block
  – first degree AV block and LBBB
- Cardiac surgery
  – aortic surgery
  – tricuspid surgery
  – ventricular septal defect closure
  – ostium primum repair

BBB, bundle branch block; LAHB, left anterior hemiblock; LPHB, left posterior hemiblock; RBBB, right bundle branch block.

---

of vascular access site complications can be reduced by using the femoral vein, with the additional advantages that haemostasis can easily be secured by pressure if bleeding occurs, and the requirement for wire manipulation during placement is usually minimal.

A sheath with a non-return valve should be placed in the vein using a Seldinger technique, to allow easy manipulation of the wire. A size 5F or 6F bipolar pacing wire is appropriate in most cases. A working pacing box (pulse generator) must be ready before inserting the wire.

When using the subclavian approach (with a standard 20–30° curve on the wire tip), the wire is advanced into the right atrium under fluoroscopic control and rotated until it points downwards and to the patient's left. Advancing across the tricuspid valve will often induce ventricular ectopics, which usually settle rapidly and require no treatment. If difficulty is encountered in crossing the tricuspid valve, changing the curve at the wire tip usually helps. If this fails, fashioning the electrode into a loop in the right atrium by pointing the lead tip to the right cardiac border may be successful. The electrode is twisted clockwise or anticlockwise until the tip lies near the tricuspid valve. Slight withdrawal of the electrode at this stage will allow the tip to flick through the valve into the right ventricle. The electrode should never be advanced if resistance is encountered; rather, the electrode should be withdrawn slightly, rotated and then advanced again. When using the femoral approach, the curve on the wire tip should be directed towards the midline as the wire enters the right atrium. As the wire is subsequently advanced it usually easily crosses the tricuspid valve.

The best position for the pacing wire is usually with the tip in the right ventricular apex, to the left of the midline and with the tip of the wire pointing inferiorly on screening (if the wire is directed to the left, towards the left shoulder, it may be in the coronary sinus and often will not capture at an acceptable threshold). There should be enough slack in the loop of the electrode to allow for changes in posture and deep inspiration, but not too much as to allow the tip to displace either in the right atrium or the pulmonary artery. The wire is then attached to the connecting leads and pacing box.

To test the threshold, the pacing box is first set to the demand mode, then the pacing rate set at 5–10 b.p.m. faster than the patient's intrinsic rate. The output is set at 3 V; this should result in a paced rhythm. The amplitude of the voltage is slowly turned down until capture is lost. Acceptable stimulation thresholds are below 1 V, although higher levels may be acceptable if the patient is elderly, has had an inferior infarct, or if several sites have been tried, all with relatively high thresholds. The stability of the pacing wire is checked during deep breathing, coughing and sniffing. If capture is lost then a more stable position should be sought. Once the threshold has been ascertained, the output voltage should be set at three times the threshold to compensate for subsequent threshold elevations due to inflammation and oedema at the electrode–tissue interface. If in sinus rhythm, a back-up rate of 50/min is set. If there is heart block or bradycardia, the rate is set at 70–80/min.

The wire is sutured firmly with a loop formed on the chest wall to minimize the chance of inadvertent lead displacement. Finally, a chest x-ray is obtained to exclude any complications.

Temporary venous pacemakers should be checked at least once daily for pacing threshold, evidence of infections around venous access sites, integrity of connections, and battery status of the external generator. Underlying rhythm should also be assessed and recorded at these checks. Pacing thresholds are checked by increasing the pacing rate to obtain continuous pacing, then progressively decreasing the output voltage until capture is lost. A sudden increase in the threshold usually indicates the need for repositioning.

Arrhythmia algorithms

VF/pulseless VT algorithm

This is recognized on the cardiac monitor by the presence of chaotic fibrillation waves, due to wandering cardiac electrical activity along continuously changing pathways (Figure 3.4a, Box 3.1) or a broad complex tachycardia (Figure 3.4b). Defibrillation with a direct current shock is the definitive treatment for VF (Figure 3.5). The likelihood of survival decreases 10 per cent for each minute of time after the onset of uncorrected VF. Defibrillation should be performed as soon as the diagnosis of VF is considered, with an initial shock of 200 J, followed by further shocks of 200 J and 360 J, if a stabilized rhythm has not been achieved. The aim is to deliver all three shocks in less than a minute. After each shock or sequence of three shocks is delivered, a pulse should be palpated only if the rhythm changes to one capable of supporting the circulation. If there is a supporting rhythm but a pulse is not palpable (pulseless electrical activity), CPR is continued for a further 1 minute, followed by a pulse check. If pulseless electrical activity persists, the non-VF/VT algorithm is followed. If VF persists, CPR is maintained for 1 minute, followed by further shocks each of 360 J (Figure 3.5). During CPR, an adequate airway and oxygenation (intubating the patient only if trained or experienced) are ensured, intravenous access obtained, and adrenaline 1 mg administered. Adrenaline is given every 3 minutes and works principally as a vasoconstrictor (alpha-agonist effect) to increase the efficiency of basic life support, not as an adjuvant to defibrillation. Adrenaline 2–3 mg (made up to a volume of 10 mL using sterile water) can be given via the tracheal tube. This should then be followed by at least five ventilations to disperse the drug into the peripheral bronchial tree and aid absorption.

At present, there is insufficient evidence to make firm recommendations on the use of any anti-arrhythmic agent for the treatment of VF/VT.

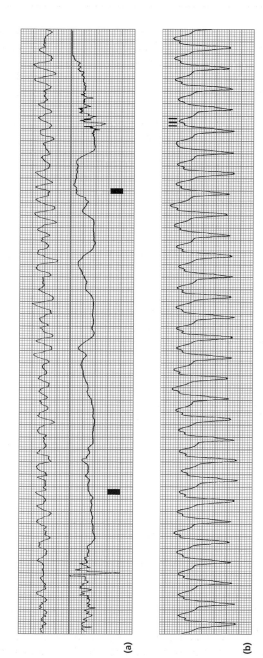

Figure 3.4 (a) Chaotic electrical activity of ventricular fibrillation. (b) Monomorphic VT: a rapid regular broad complex tachycardia.

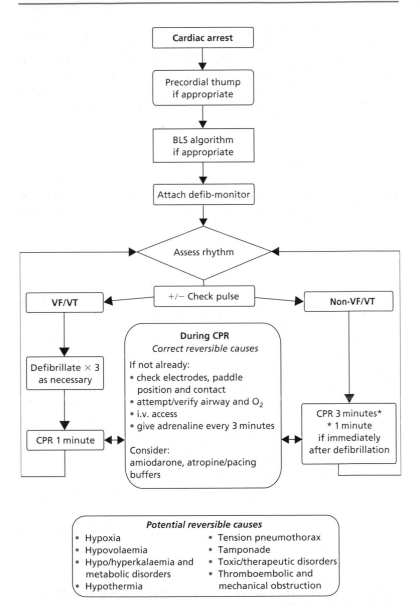

Figure 3.5 Cardiac arrest algorithm based on the European Resuscitation Council and the Resuscitation Council (UK).

Despite the lack of evidence, lignocaine has been traditionally recommended as adjuvant drug therapy for shock-resistant VF. However, recent studies suggest that amiodarone may be superior to lignocaine in cardioverting shock-resistant VF. Therefore, it is now recommended that amiodarone be used as the first-choice antifibrillatory agent. Lignocaine or procainamide can be used if amiodarone is not available. Drug doses and infusion regimens are discussed in Appendix A.

Non-VF/VT rhythms

These rhythms usually have a poor outcome unless a reversible cause can be found and rapidly treated. The right side of the resuscitation algorithm (Figure 3.5) should be followed.

Asystole

This is recognized by the total absence of any ventricular electrical activity on the cardiac monitor. Causes are summarized in Box 3.1. The gain setting on the monitor is set to 1 mV and the leads and electrical connections are secured. Where possible, an additional lead should be viewed so as to avoid missing a potentially reversible arrhythmia (fine ventricular fibrillation). If in doubt, treatment is with defibrillation as in VF/pulseless VT. Basic life support should be commenced for 3 minutes, during which time advanced airway and ventilation techniques are performed, intravenous access gained and adrenaline 1 mg given. Atropine 3 mg IV or 6 mg via the tracheal tube (made up to a volume of at least 10 mL of sterile water) is administered. The monitor should be closely inspected for the presence of atrial activity (P waves), which may suggest complete heart block with ventricular asystole. This may respond to external (transcutaneous) or transvenous pacing depending on the skills and equipment available. If asystole persists, CPR is continued with the administration of adrenaline 1 mg every 3 minutes. The administration of higher dose adrenaline as a single bolus is no longer recommended.

Pulseless electrical activity (PEA)/electromechanical dissociation (EMD)

This is recognized by the presence of an ECG rhythm compatible with a cardiac output in the setting of a cardiac arrest. The commonest cause of sudden, unexpected development of pulseless electrical activity follow-ing an acute MI is rupture of the ventricular free wall. Successful resusci-tation in this situation is very rare. Other important causes to consider are summarized in Box 3.1. The best chance of survival is the early diagnosis and treatment of the conditions detailed in Box 3.1. Having instituted basic and advanced life support, and administered any specific therapy for the above conditions, IV adrenaline 1 mg is given every 3 minutes.

Early post-resuscitation care

Immediately after an arrest, blood gases, electrolytes, cardiac specific enzymes, full blood count, ECG are checked, and any problems treated. For instance:

- Hypoxia is usually present, so high concentrations of oxygen should be given. Oxygen saturation is monitored with pulse oximetry, ensur-ing a saturation of >93 per cent.
- Serum potassium is maintained above 4 mmol/L and magnesium above 2 mmol/L. If potassium is above 6 mmol/L, 10 mL of 10 per cent calcium chloride is given IV over 5 minutes, followed by 50 mL of 50 per cent dextrose and 10 units of Actrapid (insulin) to stabilize the myocardium and correct hyperkalemia.
- If the pH is less than 7.1 or the base excess ≤ −10 mmol/L, giving bicarbonate (8.4 per cent) in 25 ml boluses should be considered to maintain a pH of 7.3–7.5.
- Starting antiarrhythmic drugs should be continued or considered.
- Hyperglycaemia should be controlled with an insulin sliding-scale regimen.
- Any persistent cardiac ischaemia that may have precipitated the cardiac arrest should be looked for and treated.
- A portable chest x-ray should be arranged and any pneumothorax treated.
- Left ventricular failure and hypotension should be treated, if pre-sent. If hypotension persists, a pulmonary artery catheter to guide optimal fluid and inotropic therapy should be considered.
- The patient should be catheterized and urine output monitored.
- The nervous system should be examined and neurological function documented using the Glasgow Coma Scale.
- The patient should be examined to ensure that there is no other med-ical or surgical intervention requiring immediate management.
- A comprehensive history should be obtained, including a family history from available witnesses. The possibility of overdoses and

other non-primary cardiac disease (such as hypothermia, cerebro-vascular accidents, subarachnoid haemorrhages, etc., see Box 3.1) should be excluded.

There are no definitive data as to when to discontinue intravenous antiarrhythmic drug infusions. It is common clinical practice to continue the infusion for a minimal of 24–48 hours and to discontinue the infusion provided there is no arrhythmic recurrence. For patients with refractory ventricular arrhythmias, high dose beta-blockade coupled with atrial or dual chamber pacemaker therapy, and light anaesthesia together with muscle relaxation and artificial ventilation, may be life saving. Urgent referral for coronary revascularization, electrophysiological testing or implantable cardioverter defibrillator insertion should be considered.

Following a successful resuscitation, most patients will regain consciousness rapidly. Hypoxia must be avoided after resuscitation, and assisted ventilation should be used if there is a reasonable chance of recovery. The patient who remains unconscious and dependent on assisted ventilation should be transferred to the intensive care unit after close liaison with the anaesthetist. The decision to withdraw ventilatory support should be made by the most senior member of the medical/anaesthetic team. The opinions of other members of the medical and nursing team, the patient (if previously known), and their relatives should be taken into consideration before making a final decision.

If asystole or PEA persists after 25 minutes of resuscitation in a normothermic adult without drug toxicity, then success is unlikely and the attempt should probably be abandoned. If VF persists at this point, the situation is still potentially reversible, and it may be worth persisting with attempts at resuscitation. Pupillary dilatation should not be used as a reason for discontinuing resuscitation, as this can be drug induced. When hypothermia is present, attempts to revive the patient should be continued for longer, probably until core temperature is above 36°C and arterial pH and potassium are normal. It is well documented that full recovery can occur with resuscitation attempts of up to 9 hours.

Late post-resuscitation care

Following a cardiac arrest, patients should be thoroughly investigated and appropriate therapy directed to minimize the risk of recurrence (Box 3.1). Reversible triggers such as acute MI, electrolyte disturbances, drugs (both prescribed and illicit) should be excluded. These can usually be diagnosed from the history, biochemical tests (including toxicology screens and cardiac specific isoenzymes) and serial ECGs. Structural heart disease can be excluded with echocardiograms, left and right heart cardiac catheterization (including right ventriculogram and myocardial biopsy) and magnetic resonance imaging (MRI). Patients with structurally normal hearts should be investigated with a 24–48-hour Holter monitor, exercise stress testing and possible programmed electrophysiological stimulation. Particular attention should be paid to the response of the QT interval during Holter monitoring and stress testing. If no triggering events can be identified, then patients should be considered for an implantable cardioverter defibrillator.

Where there is a family history of sudden cardiac death, the patient's family should be screened with an ECG, Holter monitor, echocardiogram and stress testing. Genetic screening for some of the inherited syndromes can also be carried out in some centres.

New developments

Alternative techniques to standard manual CPR have been developed to improve perfusion during CPR. Promising therapies in this regard include interposed abdominal compression CPR (IAC-CPR), and active and compression–decompression CPR (ACD-CPR). IAC-CPR requires a third rescuer and involves compression of the abdomen during the relaxation phase of chest compression. This technique appears to be equivalent or superior to standard CPR and is recommended as an alternative for professional rescuers. ACD-CPR is performed with a hand-held device equipped with suction cup to actively lift the anterior chest during decompression. This decreases intrathoracic pressure, enhancing venous return for the next compression. Randomized studies have shown equivocal benefit using this technique, and therefore it is not recommended at present.

The major determinant of survival in patients with VF and pulseless VT is the time taken for defibrillation. Consequently, there has been a natural progression to make defibrillators more available. The development and easy applicability of automatic external defibrillators have strengthened this view. Once a cardiac arrest has been diagnosed, the electrodes of the system are attached to the chest using the standard positions. The device is able to recognize VF and deliver defibrillatory shocks if required. Instructions are provided automatically on the screen and some models reinforce these instructions with synthesized voice messages. An override facility is available if one wants to use it as a manual defibrillator. These devices can be used by the public and require minimal training. Consequently, in some countries, these devices are now deployed in public locations such as airports, commercial aeroplanes, train stations and casinos. Recently, the US Food and Drug Administration have approved a vest-like defibrillator device that can be worn under clothing, rather than being implanted in the chest. The vest contains an electrode belt that is applied to the chest and monitors the heart rhythm. If an abnormal life-threatening heart rhythm is detected, and the patient loses consciousness, the device administers an electrical shock.

The conventional damped sinusoidal monophasic waveform used for defibrillation is currently being challenged by newer biphasic waveforms. If the polarity of the current is reversed part way through the delivery of a shock, the defibrillation threshold is lowered and the shock energy required for successful defibrillation is reduced. Energy requirements as low as 130 J can be used for defibrillation. Biphasic waveforms are expected to lead to the development of smaller, more portable defibrillators with the possibility of less injury to the myocardium.

Pharmacotherapy continues to evolve and although new antiarrhythmic agents are currently being evaluated, their role in resuscitation has yet to be defined. Experimentally, vasopressin, a potent vasoconstrictor, leads to significantly higher coronary perfusion pressures during CPR. It has a half-life of 10–20 minutes, which is longer than adrenaline. Preliminary data in relation to return of spontaneous circulation rates are encouraging; however, long-term outcome data are awaited before a firm recommendation can be made regarding its use during CPR.

Key points

- CPR is a dynamic subject and therefore all healthcare staff involved in patient care should be trained and kept up to date with advanced life support protocols.
- The most commonly encountered rhythm during a cardiac arrest is ventricular fibrillation or pulseless VT.
- The prognosis is less favourable for non-VF/VT rhythms unless a reversible cause is present.
- The only interventions that have been shown to improve long-term survival are basic life support and early defibrillation.
- Careful post-resuscitation care is essential to maximize the chances of a full recovery.

Key references

Adgey AAJ, Johnston PW. Approaches to modern management of cardiac arrest. *Heart* 1998; **80**: 397–401.

Eisenberg MS, Mengert TJ. Cardiac resuscitation. *N Engl J Med* 2001; **344**: 1304–13.

Gammage MD. Temporary cardiac pacing. *Heart* 2000; **83**: 715–20.

Gilbert M, Busund R, Skagseth A, Nilsen P, Solbo JP. Resuscitation from accidental hypothermia of 13.7°C with circulatory arrest. *Lancet* 2000; **355**: 375–6.

Kern KB. Cardiopulmonary resuscitation physiology. *ACC Curr J Rev* 1997; **6**: 11–13.

Kudenchuk PJ, Cobb LA, Copass MK *et al*. Amiodarone for resuscitation after out of hospital cardiac arrest due to ventricular fibrillation. *N Engl J Med* 1999; **341**: 871–8.

Nademanee K, Taylor R, Bailey WE, Rieders DE, Kosar EM. Treating electrical storm sympathetic blockade versus advanced cardiac life support-guided therapy. *Circulation* 2000; **102**: 742–7.

Peckova M, Fahrenbruch CE, Cobb LA, Hallstrom AP. Circadian variations in the occurrence of cardiac arrest. Initial and repeat episodes. *Circulation* 1998; **98**: 31–9.

Resuscitation Council (UK). *Advanced Life Support Course Provider Manual*, 4th edn. London: Resuscitation Council, 2000.

Arrhythmias

4

Background

The management of cardiac arrhythmias complicating acute myocardial infarction (MI) is dealt with in Chapter 1. This chapter deals with the management of arrhythmias that occur as a complication of other cardiac and medical disorders. Optimal treatment of these arrhythmias depends on two principles:

- inspecting the electrocardiogram (ECG) and reviewing the clinical presentation to establish the diagnosis. This provides information about arrhythmia mechanism and guides treatment selection.
- assessing the effect of the arrhythmia. Patients with good cardiac function will often tolerate arrhythmias without major haemodynamic compromise. Patients with coexistent cardiac impairment may be severely compromised by an arrhythmia. Tachyarrhythmias associated with major haemodynamic compromise usually require urgent cardioversion. Bradyarrhythmias associated with major

haemodynamic compromise often require pacing. Patients with better tolerated arrhythmias can be treated with drug therapy.

If there is any doubt about diagnosis or treatment, a senior colleague should be consulted for advice.

The symptoms produced by the onset of an arrhythmia are highly variable. In an individual with no cardiac disease, an arrhythmia may be asymptomatic. A rapid tachyarrhythmia often produces palpitations. In patients with cardiac disease, arrhythmia-related reduction in cardiac output and coronary perfusion may lead to ischaemic chest pain, heart failure and disturbed consciousness.

Supraventricular tachyarrhythmias arise from above the level of the bundle of His. Supraventricular tachyarrhythmias can be divided into two groups, depending on whether they arise from the atrial myocardium [atrial fibrillation (AF), atrial flutter and atrial tachycardia] or a mechanism involving the atrioventricular (AV) node [atrioventricular nodal re-entry tachycardia (AVNRT) and accessory pathway tachycardias]. The most common types of supraventricular tachyarrhythmia are AF and AVNRT. In the majority of patients with a supraventricular arrhythmia, ventricular activation occurs via the normal conduction system, and the arrhythmia will have a narrow QRS configuration. In a minority of patients with a supraventricular tachyarrhythmia (those with pre-existing or rate-related bundle branch block, and some patients with an accessory pathway), abnormal slow ventricular activation occurs, and the arrhythmia will have a broad complex QRS configuration. Ventricular tachyarrhythmias arise below the AV node and almost always have a broad QRS configuration (although some that arise high in the bundle of His can be relatively narrow). Because of this overlap, QRS duration is not a totally reliable guide to the site of origin of an arrhythmia, and additional information obtained from careful inspection of all features of the ECG is required before a diagnosis can be reached.

Antiarrhythmic drug therapy has important limitations. The available agents are of limited efficacy, and a drug prescribed in the correct dose for an appropriate indication may fail to work. The available drugs have many unwanted side effects, commonly causing gastrointestinal and central nervous system disturbances, impairment of cardiovascular function or pro-arrhythmia. The available drugs can be categorized using the Vaughan–Williams classification, which provides information on the drugs' electrophysiological effects:

- CLASS I: these agents have membrane-stabilizing properties, slowing sodium transport during myocyte depolarization, and can act on the atria, ventricles or conduction tissue.

- CLASS II: these agents block cardiac beta-receptors and act predominantly on the sinus and AV nodes (although there is also some membrane-stabilizing effect in the atria and ventricles).
- CLASS III: these agents act on myocyte potassium channels, prolong the duration of the action potential and can act on the atria, ventricles or conduction system.
- CLASS IV: these agents block calcium channels, and act predominantly on the sinus and AV nodes.

Some drugs have more than one class of action, and others such as adenosine and digoxin cannot be classified using this simple system. Because of the complex nature of these drugs and the potential to induce a wide range of adverse effects, it is important to become familiar with the use of a small number of front-line drugs. Polypharmacy should be avoided; if the first-line therapy fails, a senior colleague should be contacted for advice before using a second drug. The onset of an arrhythmia is often associated with associated problems such as heart failure, pulmonary infection or embolism, thyroid disturbance, hypoxia, electrolyte imbalance or drug administration. It is important to look for and treat correctable factors that may initiate or perpetuate an arrhythmia.

Atrial fibrillation

Background

Atrial fibrillation (AF) is the most common cardiac arrhythmia (Figure 4.1). The incidence of AF rises with age, and it is very common in the elderly population (affecting 10 per cent of people over the age of 70). The development of AF is associated with atrial electrical instability or atrial distension induced by:

- ischaemic heart disease
- hypertension
- valvular heart disease
- heart failure
- pulmonary infection or embolism.

Other less common causes of AF are cardiac trauma (including iatrogenic trauma associated with cardiac surgery), metabolic abnormalities, exposure to toxins (such as alcohol), pericardial disease or systemic infection. In some patients, AF can arise in an otherwise entirely normal heart. This lone AF may be due to small localized areas of electrical instability in the atrium (usually close to the pulmonary vein orifices),

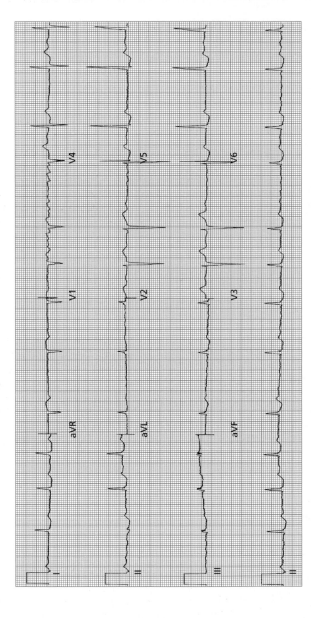

Figure 4.1 Atrial fibrillation is characterized by the absence of P waves and an irregular ventricular rhythm. The 'reverse tick' deformity of the ST segment, associated with digoxin, is best seen here in leads V5 and V6.

or increased susceptibility to fluctuations in autonomic neural stimuli to the heart.

Diagnosis and assessment

Regardless of the underlying aetiology, patients with AF develop multiple random wavelets of depolarization in the atrial myocardium. This rapid erratic electrical activity is intermittently conducted to the ventricles via the AV node, producing a rapid, irregularly irregular ventricular rhythm. The onset of AF is often associated with symptoms due to a reduction in cardiac output or the rapid irregular ventricular rhythm causing a sensation of palpitation. The mean resting rate in patients with new onset AF is usually between 110 and 130 b.p.m. A rate in excess of 150 b.p.m. should raise the suspicion of a hyperadrenergic state (thyrotoxicosis, or fever) or acute blood loss. A very rapid (rate 250 b.p.m.) broad complex AF is suggestive of the presence of a rapidly conducting accessory pathway.

When AF persists for more than 48 hours, stasis of blood in the fibrillating atrium may lead to clot formation and systemic embolization. The risk of thromboembolism is low in patients with recent onset (up to 48 hours' duration) AF. In some patients (particularly if cardiac function is normal) the AF will be well tolerated and asymptomatic. The 12-lead ECG of patients with AF will show an absence of P waves, rapid erratic fibrillation activity visible in the baseline between ventricular complexes and an irregularly irregular ventricular rhythm which usually has a narrow complex QRS configuration. Initially, episodes of AF may be short-lived and self-terminating (paroxysmal AF). Repeated episodes, however, lead to adverse changes in atrial electrophysiological and mechanical function, which decrease electrical stability and eventually lead to the development of sustained AF. Episodes of AF that persist for several days rarely terminate spontaneously.

In patient assessment, careful history taking and clinical examination are important. If there is time, a chest x-ray and echocardiogram will also help. Particular importance should be paid to:

- the duration of AF;
- the presence of coexistent cardiac disease (such as hypertension, ischaemic heart disease, valvular heart disease or left ventricular dysfunction);
- the effects of AF on patient symptoms, ventricular rate, blood pressure (BP) and cardiac function.

These important features help to guide the selection of appropriate therapy.

Treatment of recent-onset poorly tolerated AF

The onset of AF may be poorly tolerated, producing major symptoms and haemodynamic compromise. Patients with coexistent structural abnormalities (such as valvular heart disease, left ventricular hypertrophy, coronary artery disease or left ventricular dysfunction) or an accessory pathway capable of rapid antegrade conduction are intolerant of AF. When AF is poorly tolerated, many antiarrhythmic drugs are contraindicated or have an unpredictable response. If AF is associated with:

- angina or heart failure,
- rate > 200 b.p.m.,
- systolic BP < 90 mmHg,

urgent restoration of sinus rhythm by direct current cardioversion (DCC) is the treatment of choice. As long as the AF is of <48 hours' duration, the risk of procedure-related thromboembolism is low. After restoration of sinus rhythm, heparinization followed by warfarin (for at least 1 month) is indicated to guard against thromboembolism if the AF recurs.

Treatment of recent-onset well tolerated AF

In patients with recent onset (<48 hours) AF who do not have major symptoms or haemodynamic instability, AF can be treated with antiarrhythmic drugs. Heparin should be commenced immediately the diagnosis is made, followed by warfarin for at least 1 month. Drugs that act predominantly on the AV node (such as digoxin, beta-blockers and calcium antagonists) are not effective at restoring sinus rhythm. Class I or class III drugs that act on the atrial myocardium can restore sinus rhythm in most patients if the drugs are administered early in adequate doses, with the highest success rates achieved by some class I drugs. If the patient has a structurally normal heart (no significant valve disease, ischaemic heart disease or left ventricular dysfunction) intravenous (IV) flecainide 2 mg/kg restores sinus rhythm in 90 per cent of patients within 1 hour. The use of flecainide should be avoided if there is any pre-existing structural heart disease, as this will increase the risk of major adverse effects. In a patient with associated structural heart disease, an IV bolus of amiodarone 300 mg followed by an infusion of 900 mg over 24 hours is safe (see Appendix A), produces rapid slowing of the ventricular rate (due to its beta-blocking effects) and is moderately effective for cardioversion. If pharmacological cardioversion fails, DCC should be considered.

Treatment of well tolerated AF of long or unknown duration

If the AF has been present for more than 48 hours, there is a significant thromboembolic risk associated with cardioversion. If the time of onset cannot be identified, the arrhythmia duration may exceed 48 hours with an associated increase in thromboembolism risk. In these patients, a strategy of anticoagulation and ventricular rate control is required. Anticoagulation should be instituted with heparin followed by warfarin. Digoxin takes several hours to slow the ventricular rate (acting indirectly on the AV node via the autonomic nervous system) and its efficacy is reduced in a hyperadrenergic patient. Intravenous beta-blockers produce rapid rate control regardless of the level of sympathetic tone. A cardioselective agent such as atenolol 5 mg by slow IV injection is effective in most patients. If the ventricular rate remains rapid and BP is >100 mmHg, a further 2.5 mg can be given after 10 minutes, followed by a further 2.5 mg after another 2 minutes if necessary. Intravenous therapy should be followed by adequate oral doses of atenolol (50–100 mg). If there is coexistent ventricular dysfunction, digoxin (0.125–0.5 mg) is the drug of choice for long-term rate control. Cardioversion should be considered after a month's anticoagulation.

Atrial flutter

Atrial flutter is a relatively uncommon arrhythmia (Figure 4.2). The electrophysiological mechanism is different from that of AF. In most patients with atrial flutter a re-entry circuit in the right atrium depolarizes at a rate of 300/min in a circular anticlockwise direction, down the lateral border of the right atrium, through an area of slowed conduction near the tricuspid valve annulus and back up the atrial septum. The normal AV node cannot conduct at this rate, and 2:1 AV block occurs. The electrocardiogram shows a regular narrow complex tachycardia (in the absence of bundle branch block) at a rate of 150 b.p.m. This rate may be slower in a patient with impaired AV nodal function, or faster if sympathetic nervous system activation is present. Atrial activity may be visible on the ECG, seen as saw-tooth flutter waves with a rate of 300/min, best visualized in V1. The flutter waves may only be visible during a temporary increase in the degree of AV block induced by vagal manoeuvres or intravenous adenosine. Atrial flutter may degenerate into AF, or the rhythm may alternate between flutter and fibrillation.

The onset of atrial flutter may be associated with symptoms of haemodynamic compromise due to the rapid ventricular rate and loss

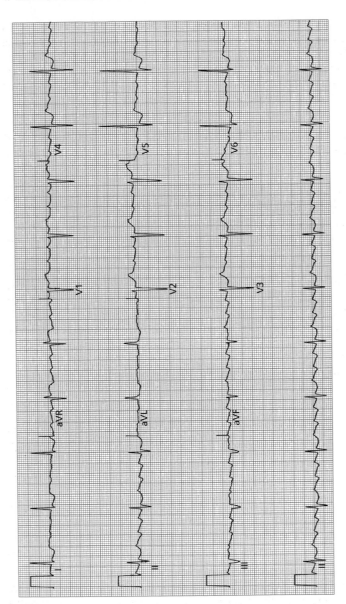

Figure 4.2 Atrial flutter is characterized by the undulating saw-tooth baseline (flutter waves) between the QRS complexes. The flutter waves are best seen in the inferior leads and lead V1. In this case the flutter rate is 250 b.p.m. and there is 4:1 AV block.

of effective atrial mechanical activity. There is a risk of clot formation in the atria in atrial flutter, leading to systemic embolism, and these patients require appropriate antithrombotic therapy as well as arrhythmia treatment. Attempts to slow the ventricular rate using drugs are often unsuccessful, and the aim of treatment should be to restore sinus rhythm. Treatment depends on the clinical circumstances:

- If the arrhythmia is associated with significant haemodynamic compromise (systolic BP < 90 mmHg), or symptoms of angina, impaired conscious level or heart failure, urgent DCC is the treatment of choice.
- If the arrhythmia is well tolerated, an attempt can be made to restore sinus rhythm with drug therapy. Atrial flutter is often resistant to treatment with drugs. Class I antiarrhythmic drugs may terminate atrial flutter, but can also cause a poorly tolerated increase in ventricular rate (by slowing the flutter rate to less than 300/min and therefore facilitating 1:1 atrioventricular conduction at a rate greater than 150 b.p.m.). Amiodarone has beneficial effects on atrial electrical stability, and may terminate the arrhythmia. In addition, amiodarone impairs atrioventricular conduction, and this property will help to slow the ventricular rate. We therefore recommend IV amiodarone for the treatment of atrial flutter, using the regimen detailed in Appendix A. If amiodarone is ineffective, the ventricular rate can be slowed with IV atenolol 5–10 mg. Anticoagulation and cardioversion can then be performed following the same guidelines as for AF. Although atrial flutter is a relatively organized rhythm and thrombus formation is less likely to occur, anticoagulation should be used as in atrial fibrillation, particularly if other risk factors (such as marked atrial enlargement or mitral valve disease) are present.
- Overdrive pacing is an alternative treatment that is effective in restoring sinus rhythm in 70 per cent of patients. If facilities are available, a temporary pacing wire is positioned against the lateral wall of the right atrium. A burst of rapid atrial pacing at a rate of 400 b.p.m. for several seconds will usually restore sinus rhythm. Occasionally AF will be precipitated, and this will often spontaneously revert to sinus rhythm. If it persists, it is easier to treat than atrial flutter.
- If atrial flutter persists despite 24 hours of intravenous amiodarone, or is resistant to overdrive pacing, DCC (often at very low energies) has a high success rate in restoring sinus rhythm.

Chronic drug therapy of atrial flutter has only limited efficacy. Radio-frequency ablation (with targeted lesions around the tricuspid annulus designed to interrupt the macro re-entry circuit) has much better success rates (up to 97 per cent in some cases) and is preferable for suitable patients.

Atrioventricular nodal re-entry tachycardia (AVNRT)

Background

Atrioventricular nodal re-entry is the mechanism responsible for most (70 per cent) episodes of symptomatic paroxysmal regular narrow complex tachycardia. This is a common arrhythmia, associated with recurrent attacks of palpitation throughout life, usually with an onset between 30 and 50 years of age. It is more common in women than men. In most patients there is no associated valvular, myocardial or coronary artery disease. Tachycardia onset is associated with sudden onset of rapid palpitation, which may be associated with dizziness, syncope and polyuria. The arrhythmia is usually well tolerated haemodynamically, because the heart is structurally normal. In patients with the common form of AVNRT, the AV node has two functionally and anatomically distinct pathways. These two pathways are joined into a final common pathway through the lower part of the AV node. One pathway is capable of fast conduction, and conducts electrical activity from atria to ventricles in normal sinus rhythm. The other pathway is slow conducting and is redundant during normal sinus rhythm. This slow pathway, however, has a short refractory period, and recovers its ability to conduct before the fast pathway. An appropriately timed atrial ectopic can be conducted down the slow pathway and back up the fast pathway, setting up a regular continuously reciprocating mechanism responsible for the sudden onset of a tachycardia. This re-entry in the AV node depolarizes atria and ventricles simultaneously, and resultant P waves are not visible because they are superimposed on the QRS complex. The ECG therefore shows a rapid regular narrow complex tachycardia (in the absence of bundle branch block) with a rate between 130 and 250 b.p.m. and no visible P waves. The heart rate varies with activity of the autonomic nervous system, increasing in association with sympathetic activation (for example standing up increases sympathetic activation, speeding up AV nodal conduction and increasing the tachycardia rate). The tachycardia can induce ST segment and T-wave changes that persist for some time after termination of the arrhythmia, but the ECG is usually normal between attacks.

Treatment

Most episodes of AVNRT can be terminated by vagal manoeuvres or intravenous drug therapy. Stimulating the vagus by a Valsalva manoeuvre, carotid sinus massage or activation of the diving reflex (by application of a cold stimulus to the face) will temporarily slow AV nodal conduction and interrupt the tachycardia circuit, terminating the arrhythmia in some patients. Some of these techniques can be used by the patient to try and terminate an attack at home, avoiding the need to attend hospital. Adenosine has a very short half-life (as short as 1.5 seconds), no significant haemodynamic side effects, and is very effective at terminating AVNRT. Adenosine is given as a rapid bolus at 3 mg into a peripheral vein, immediately flushed through with 10 mL saline. If this fails, incremental doses of 6 mg, 9 mg and 12 mg should be administered. Transient facial flushing, dyspnoea and chest pain are common, but last for less than 20 seconds.

Adenosine can induce bronchospasm and is contraindicated in patients with asthma or AV block. It should also be used with caution in patients with chronic obstructive pulmonary disease (COPD) because of the potential to induce or exacerbate bronchospasm. If drug-induced bronchospasm occurs, further drug administration should be withheld and, if necessary, treatment with nebulized bronchodilators commenced. Dipyridamole potentiates the effects of adenosine, and dosage should be reduced to an initial 1 mg, increasing to a maximum of 4 mg if required. Theophyllines antagonize the action of adenosine, which may render the drug ineffective in these patients.

If adenosine is contraindicated or ineffective, verapamil is an effective alternative agent, given as 5–10 mg over 30–60 seconds. Verapamil should be avoided if:

- systolic BP is <100 mmHg;
- left ventricular function is known to be impaired;
- QRS complex is >120 ms (three small squares);
- patient is receiving concurrent treatment with beta-blockers;
- patient is known to have an accessory pathway.

If both adenosine and verapamil are contraindicated, a senior colleague should be consulted; the options would be to use a class I antiarrhythmic drug, or pace termination. To terminate AVNRT by pacing:

- A temporary pacing wire is placed in contact with the atrial endocardium and pacing instituted at 100 b.p.m. If a pacing spike occurs at an appropriate time point it will induce a critical refractory period in the circuit and terminate the arrhythmia.
- If underdrive pacing fails, the atria is paced 20 per cent faster than the tachycardia rate for 30 seconds, then the pacing abruptly terminated. This will often terminate the arrhythmia by a similar mechanism to underdrive pacing. There is a small risk of precipitating AF, which is usually short-lived and reverts to sinus rhythm.

If all these measures fail, DCC can be used to restore sinus rhythm.

Accessory pathway tachycardias

Background

In the normal heart the atria and ventricles become electrically isolated during fetal development. The only route by which atrial electrical activity can be conducted to the ventricles is via the AV node. Incomplete separation of the atria and ventricles during fetal development leads to the persistence of a connection that is capable of abnormally conducting electrical activity between atria and ventricles. These abnormal connections are called accessory pathways, and they can be responsible for a variety of ECG abnormalities and tachyarrhythmias. Accessory pathways are the mechanism responsible for around 20 per cent of paroxysmal regular supraventricular tachyarrhythmias. The pathways can arise in a variety of different sites around the AV rings, and connect to various areas of the ventricles or conduction system. The most common position for an accessory pathway is in the left lateral free wall of the heart. Less commonly, pathways can be situated close to the septum, in the right free wall, or, rarely, can be multiple. The appearance of the surface ECG and the type of arrhythmias that occur depend on the precise anatomy and conduction characteristics of the accessory pathway. Accessory pathway tachycardias are more common in males than females. The commonest arrhythmia in these patients arises when electrical activity repeatedly circulates between the atria and ventricles via the AV node and accessory pathway, producing an atrioventricular re-entry tachycardia (AVRT). Atrial fibrillation is a less common but potentially dangerous arrhythmia (if AF occurs in a patient with a pathway that is capable of rapid antegrade conduction from atria to ventricles, rapid stimulation of the ventricles can result in VF and sudden cardiac death).

Diagnosis from the ECG during sinus rhythm

In many patients with an accessory pathway, the resting ECG will be abnormal. If the pathway is capable of antegrade conduction from atria to ventricles, initial slow ventricular activation will occur via the pathway during normal sinus rhythm. This produces a short PR interval and delta wave (Figure 4.3). This type of accessory pathway is present in up to 3 per 1000 of the population (although many of these patients never have symptoms). The occurrence of arrhythmias in association with this type of pathway and abnormal ECG is termed Wolff–Parkinson–White (WPW) syndrome. The common left-sided pathways produce a

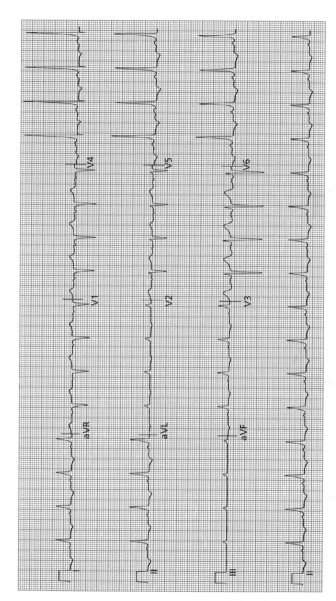

Figure 4.3 Wolff–Parkinson–White syndrome. A short PR interval and delta waves indicate the presence of an accessory pathway.

predominantly positive QRS complex in V1. The less common right-sided pathways produce a predominantly negative QRS complex in V1. In some patients the accessory pathway is only capable of retrograde conduction from ventricles to atria. In these patients ventricular activation occurs normally via the AV node, there is no pre-excitation, and the surface ECG during sinus rhythm is completely normal. This 'concealed' accessory pathway is, however, still capable of conducting retrogradely, thereby participating in the re-entry circuit of an AVRT. The presence of a concealed accessory pathway is suggested by the characteristics of the ECG during tachycardia, indicating AV re-entry as a possible tachycardia mechanism.

Atrioventricular re-entry tachycardia (AVRT)

Because the AV node and accessory pathway have different refractory periods, an appropriately timed ectopic can initiate a repetitive cycle of depolarization involving the AV node and accessory pathway. In the common type of AVRT, electrical activity passes to the ventricles via the AV node, then back via the accessory pathway to depolarize the atria and re-initiate the cycle (orthodromic tachycardia). Since ventricular depolarization occurs via the normal conduction system, the ECG will show a rapid regular narrow complex tachycardia (with no pre-excitation). Since atrial depolarization occurs after ventricular depolarization, an inverted P wave may be visible roughly halfway between QRS complexes. Rarely, activation passes from atria to ventricles via an antegradely conducting pathway, then back to the atria via the AV node. Since ventricular depolarization is initiated via the pathway, the tachycardia will have a broad QRS morphology (antidromic tachycardia). This type of rare AVRT is difficult to differentiate from ventricular tachycardia (VT) without the aid of an electrophysiological study (EPS).

Atrial fibrillation (AF)

AF is less common in patients with accessory pathways, but can be life threatening. The atria depolarize rapidly (350–600 impulses per minute) during AF. In a normal individual, the AV node protects the ventricles from this rapid erratic electrical activity. If AF occurs in a patient with an accessory pathway that is capable of rapid antegrade conduction, rapid atrial electrical activity can be conducted directly to the ventricles, resulting in a very fast ventricular response that can lead to haemo-dynamic collapse, or degenerate to VF. The ECG will show an irregularly irregular rhythm with a variable QRS morphology (due to most com-plexes being conducted via the pathway, leading to a broad QRS morph-ology, with a minority conducted via the AV node leading to a narrow QRS morphology).

Treatment

In patients with WPW sydrome who present with the common form of narrow complex orthodromic tachycardia and who are not haemo-dynamically compromised, initial drug therapy is appropriate. As a general principle, drugs that predominantly block AV nodal conduction should be avoided in patients known to have an accessory pathway. In certain circumstances, AV nodal blocking drugs can cause tachycardia acceleration (for instance in patients with AF and a pathway capable of rapid anterograde conduction). It is therefore preferable to use a drug that acts predominantly to slow accessory pathway conduction. Intra-venous flecainide 2 mg/kg has a good safety profile in a patient with an accessory pathway, and will terminate more than 80 per cent of episodes. If flecainide fails, consult a senior colleague before adminis-tering another drug. If the patient is haemodynamically compromised with the tachycardia, DCC is the treatment of choice.

When AF occurs in a patient with a pathway capable of rapid ante-grade conduction, the ventricular rate can exceed 250 b.p.m. These rapid ventricular rates are often associated with haemodynamic com-promise or heart failure, and urgent DC cardioversion is required. If the AF is slower and well tolerated, a drug that slows accessory pathway conduction (such as flecainide 2 mg/kg IV) can be used to slow the ventricular rate and restore sinus rhythm.

Because of the inherent risk of sudden death, all patients with an accessory pathway should be reviewed by an electrophysiologist to plan an optimal investigation and treatment strategy. The most danger-ous pathways are those that are capable of rapid antegrade conduction from atria to ventricles. Concealed pathways and pathways that show intermittent pre-excitation or pre-excitation that disappears with exercise are unlikely to be capable of rapid antegrade conduction, but electrophysiological characterization of the conduction characteristics of the pathway is more reliable that inspection of the surface ECG. Ablation is highly successful and low risk, and should be considered for all patients with an accessory pathway (the risks of long-term antiarrhythmic drug therapy are probably greater than the procedure-related risks of EPS and ablation).

Atrial tachycardia

Atrial tachycardia is relatively rare. Unifocal atrial tachycardia arises from a single repetitively discharging area of micro re-entry or enhanced automaticity. During the arrhythmia the ECG will usually show a regular narrow complex tachycardia with a rate of 120–240 b.p.m. (Figure 4.4). Each QRS complex will be preceded by a morphologically abnormal P wave, usually best seen in V1. An upright P wave in V1 indicates the tachycardia is due to a left atrial focus, a positive P wave in AVL indicates a right atrial origin. The arrhythmia can arise in patients with structural heart disease leading to atrial dilatation or dysfunction, but commonly no cause is found. Atrial tachycardia is often resistant to drug therapy. Nodal blocking drugs will not terminate the arrhythmia, but may slow the ventricular rate. Antiarrhythmic drugs that stabilize atrial electrical activity (such as sotalol, flecainide, and amiodarone) may terminate the arrhythmia. If drug therapy fails, overdrive pacing or cardioversion should be considered.

Unifocal atrial tachycardia may arise as a complication of digoxin toxicity. In this case, digoxin induces a variable degree of atrioventricular block as well as triggering the discharge of an atrial ectopic focus. The atrial rate is generally 150–200 b.p.m., and the degree of atrioventricular block may fluctuate, producing an irregular ventricular rhythm. When atrial tachycardia with variable block complicates digoxin therapy:

- further digoxin therapy should be withheld until the arrhythmia resolves;
- beta-blockers should be given (if necessary) to slow the ventricular rate;
- potassium should be maintained above 4.0 mmol/L;
- Digibind (see Chapter 9) should be considered.

DCC should be avoided, as it may induce intractable arrhythmias in a patient with digoxin toxicity.

Multifocal atrial tachycardia most commonly arises as a complication of respiratory disease in acutely ill elderly patients, and is characterized by multiple atrial foci producing constant variation in the P-wave morphology and a variable atrial rate (Figure 4.5). Therapy consists of ensuring that the potassium level is adequate, treating the underlying respiratory problem, and using AV nodal blocking drugs to control the ventricular rate.

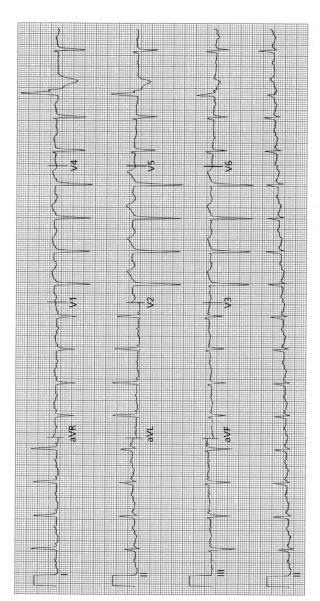

Figure 4.4 Atrial tachycardia. Note the morphologically abnormal P waves seen best in the limb leads.

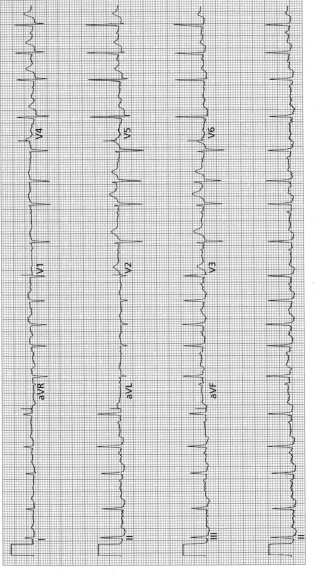

Figure 4.5 Multifocal atrial tachycardia is characterized by the following: a rate more than 100/min; organized, discrete non-sinus P waves with at least three different forms in the same ECG lead; isoelectric baseline between P waves; and irregular PP, PR and RR intervals. In patients with heart rates less than 100/min, the term multifocal atrial rhythm is used.

Ventricular arrhythmias

Background

A tachycardia with broad QRS complexes can be due to:

- ventricular tachycardia (VT);
- supraventricular tachycardia in a patient with pre-existing or rate-related bundle branch block;
- supraventricular tachycardia in a patient with an accessory pathway that is capable of antegrade conduction.

A series of clinical and ECG guidelines can be used to determine the site of tachycardia origin. The patient's general clinical state is no guide to the site of tachycardia origin. The degree of haemodynamic compromise that occurs depends on the ventricular rate and left ventricular function. A rapid supraventricular tachycardia in a patient with left ventricular dysfunction may cause major haemodynamic collapse, whilst a slow VT may be well tolerated in a patient with good left ventricular function. If the patient is not severely compromised, clinical assessment, a 12-lead ECG or the use of IV adenosine helps to identify the site of origin of a broad complex tachycardia. The useful features are:

- A totally irregular broad complex tachycardia is likely to be AF with bundle branch block or an accessory pathway.
- Capture or fusion beats, independent P waves that are dissociated from ventricular activity or clinical evidence of AV dissociation (cannon waves or variable intensity S1) confirm that the tachycardia is VT.
- A broad QRS (>140 ms), marked axis deviation, ventricular concordance, a deep S wave in V6 or an RSr pattern in V1 suggest a ventricular origin (Figure 4.6).
- If an IV adenosine bolus has no effect on the tachycardia, it is probably VT. If the arrhythmia terminates, it is probably of supraventricular origin. The transient period of AV block associated with adenosine administration may allow visualization of atrial fibrillation, flutter or tachycardia activity.

It is important to remember that most broad complex tachycardias are due to VT, particularly if the patient is known to have structural heart disease. Intravenous verapamil should never be given to a patient with a broad complex tachycardia as it may cause severe and intractable haemodynamic depression if the tachycardia is VT. If doubt as to the diagnosis remains after clinical assessment, inspection of the ECG and administration of adenosine, then the arrhythmia should be treated as VT.

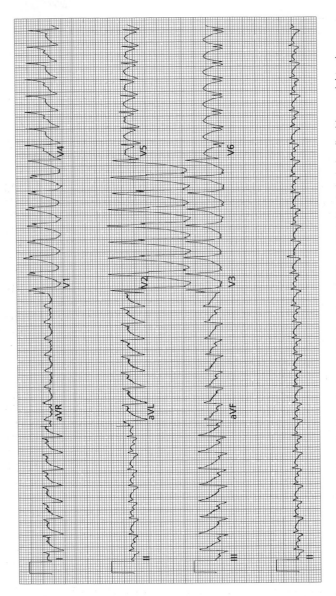

Figure 4.6 Ventricular tachycardia. Note, the broad QRS duration (>140 ms), marked axis deviation (in this case right axis deviation), RSr pattern in lead V1, deep S in lead V5 and V6, AV dissociation (best seen in lead II), and a fusion beat (nineteenth QRS complex on the rhythm strip).

Monomorphic VT

The commonest cause of monomorphic VT is ischaemic heart disease. Monomorphic VT occurring early in the course of acute MI is usually due to enhanced automaticity in the infarcting segment of myocardium. Monomorphic VT occurring late after MI is usually associated with re-entry in scar tissue. Less common causes include cardiomyopathy, myocarditis, arrhythmogenic right ventricular dysplasia, valvular heart disease, or scarring associated with cardiac surgery. Occasionally, monomorphic VT can arise in an entirely normal heart. The occurrence of monomorphic VT with a left bundle and right axis configuration in a patient with a normal heart indicates that the arrhythmia is arising from the right ventricular outflow tract. A relatively narrow QRS duration suggests that the origin of the tachycardia lies close to the bundle of His (fascicular VT). Both these tachycardias can be terminated by adenosine and are amenable to radiofrequency ablation. If the resting ECG shows T-wave inversion in V1–V3 and there is a family history of palpitations or sudden death, arrhythmogenic right ventricular dysplasia is a possibility. If the arrhythmia is exercise induced in a structurally normal heart, right ventricular outflow tachycardia is a possibility.

Monomorphic VT consists of a rapid succession of ventricular ectopic beats occurring at a rate >120 b.p.m. The rhythm will be predominantly regular and each successive ventricular complex will have a uniform appearance. The regularity and morphology of the tachycardia may be intermittently altered by the occurrence of capture of fusion beats. Monomorphic VT that lasts for less than 30 seconds is defined as non-sustained. A right bundle branch block configuration indicates a left ventricular origin for the tachycardia, whilst a left bundle branch block configuration indicates a right ventricular origin. Treatment of sustained monomorphic VT is detailed in Chapter 1. If the monomorphic VT is not clearly related to an acute MI, there is a high risk of recurrence, and expert investigation is required to determine the underlying cause. The investigations to consider are:

- coronary angiography to evaluate the presence and extent of coronary artery disease in patients with ischaemic heart disease;
- cardiac imaging with echocardiography or magnetic resonance imaging (MRI) scanning to evaluate cardiac structure and function in patients with cardiomyopathy;
- stress testing to look for exercise-induced ischaemia or VT;
- signal-averaged ECG to look for late potentials (which act as a substrate that can induce VT).

If an identifiable treatable precipitating factor such as cardiac ischaemia can be identified, this should be treated before using antiarrhythmic drugs. If there is no clear treatable factor, drug therapy or implantation of an autonomic implantable cardioverter defibrillator (AICD) should be considered. An AICD is preferable if the VT was associated with cardiac arrest, major haemodynamic compromise, the patient has an ejection fraction of <35 per cent or an abnormality such as cardiomyopathy is present. If the patient is not suitable for AICD implantation, drug therapy is an inferior alternative. The most effective drugs to prevent recurrence of VT are sotalol and amiodarone. After commencing chronic oral therapy, efficacy should be evaluated by EPS (to ensure non-inducibility) or ambulatory ECG (to ensure arrhythmia suppression). If either test indicates poor control, modification of drug therapy or consideration of other options such as AICD, ablation therapy or surgery is indicated.

Polymorphic VT

Polymorphic VT is characterized by repeated progressive changes in QRS morphology and orientation, producing an appearance of twisting around the baseline (Figure 4.7). Polymorphic VT in the absence of QT prolongation is mainly associated with MI, and is dealt with in Chapter 1. Polymorphic VT occurring in association with QT prolongation, is termed *torsades de pointes* tachycardia. This type of VT occurs when abnormal ventricular repolarization with resultant QT prolongation occurs due to bradycardia, hypokalaemia, hypomagnesaemia or drugs. The common drugs associated with QT prolongation are antiarrhythmics, antibiotics, antihistamines, and antipsychotics. Rarely, QT prolongation may be congenital, when it is due to inherited or sporadic genetic defects of myocyte potassium and sodium channels. Treatment consists of:

- withdrawal of any implicated drugs;
- treatment of sustained episodes with DCC if associated with haemodynamic collapse;
- pacing at 100 b.p.m. to shorten the QT interval;
- giving IV magnesium 8 mmol stat then 2.5 mmol/h infusion for 24 hours.

In patients with congenital QT prolongation, beta-blockade, sympathectomy or an AICD may be required.

Ventricular fibrillation (VF)

The commonest cause of VF is ischaemic heart disease, and it is responsible for 90 per cent of deaths caused by acute MI. The emergency management of VF is dealt with in Chapters 1 and 3. If VF occurs in the

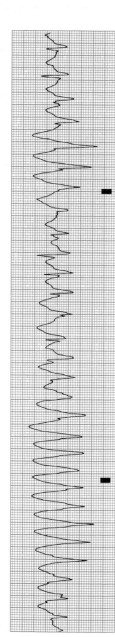

Figure 4.7 Polymorphic VT. Note the frequent changes in QRS complex morphology.

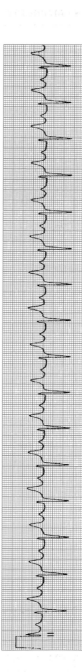

Figure 4.8 First degree AV block characterized by a PR interval >0.2 seconds.

absence of evidence of an evolving MI, careful investigation is required as described for VT. All patients who survive an episode of VF not associated with acute MI should be considered for an AICD, as this is more effective than drug therapy.

Bradyarrhythmias

Background

Bradyarrhythmias arising as a complication of acute MI (particularly inferior MI) are dealt with in Chapter 1. Bradyarrhythmias that are not related to acute MI are most commonly due to idiopathic fibrosis of the conduction system (which is more common in the elderly), although a wide range of other cardiac conditions can occasionally be responsible. These bradyarrhythmias may present with important symptoms that require urgent treatment.

Heart block

First degree heart block (prolongation of the PR interval to >0.20 seconds) signifies slow conduction of electrical activity from atria to ventricles (Figure 4.8). First degree block does not cause symptoms, and can occur in young people in association with high vagal tone. In older individuals it may indicate the presence of underlying fibrosis in the conduction system with a risk of progression to higher grade AV block. In second degree block there is intermittent failure of conduction of atrial impulses to the ventricles, manifest as P wave not followed by a QRS complex. In Mobitz type I (Wenkebach) second degree AV block, a progressive increase in impaired conduction in the AV node occurs with each successive sinus beat. This leads to a progressive prolongation in the PR interval until an atrial impulse fails to be conducted, resulting in a dropped beat. After the dropped beat, AV conduction recovers and the sequence is repeated. Mobtiz type I block can be a benign phenomenon occurring in normal individuals with high vagal tone, particularly during sleep. In the absence of high vagal tone in a younger individual, Mobitz type I block is associated with a significant risk of progression to high degree AV block with symptoms. In Mobitz type II second degree AV block, impaired conduction in the bundle of His or bundle branches leads to intermittent failure of conduction of atrial impulses to the ventricles without preceding lengthening of the PR interval. These patients often have associated bundle branch block and axis deviation (bifascicular block), occasionally with associated PR interval prolongation, reflecting extensive disease in the bundle of His. Patients with Mobitz type II block have extensive conduction system disease and are at increased risk of Stokes–Adams attacks, slow ventricular rates and sudden death. Complete heart block occurs when there is total failure of conduction of electrical activity from atria to ventricles (Figure 4.9). Complete heart block can be due to disease at nodal or bundle of His level. If the block is at nodal level, the escape rhythm that results will be narrow complex, stable, and usually fast enough to support an adequate circulation. In patients with extensive disease in the bundle of His, the subsidiary pacemaker will be low in the conduction system, producing a slow, unreliable broad complex escape rhythm, with an increased risk of major symptoms. When fibrosis predominantly affects the sinus node and atria, sick sinus syndrome occurs. This is characterized by a variety of often intermittent tachy- or bradyarrhythmias. The common rhythm disturbances are:

- sinus bradycardia
- sinus arrest
- atrial flutter or fibrillation.

In up to one-third of these patients the fibrotic process extends into the AV node and heart block coexists.

Clinical features and management

The electrocardiographic features of heart block are discussed in Chapter 1. In sick sinus syndrome the ECG shows sinus bradycardia, sinus arrest, atrial fibrillation or flutter and sometimes AV block (these features may only be evident with prolonged rhythm monitoring). First degree and Mobitz type I AV block do not cause symptoms. If the conduction disturbance is not clearly associated with high vagal tone, close monitoring is required as higher grade AV block may develop. In patients with bifascicular block, there is a small risk of progression to complete heart block, but pacing in the absence of symptoms is not required. If general anaesthesia is required for non-cardiac surgery in a patient with bifascicular block and prolongation of the PR interval, many authorities recommend prophylactic temporary pacing to guard against sudden complete heart block.

In Mobitz type II and complete heart block a slow ventricular rate may cause tiredness, dyspnoea, or heart failure. If the escape rhythm is unreliable or intermittently fails, syncope or sudden death may occur.

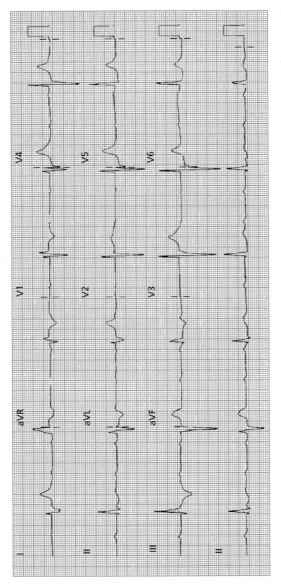

Figure 4.9 Complete heart block. There is complete AV dissociation with the P waves and QRS complexes occurring without any relation to each other. Note the constantly changing PR intervals.

Patients with sick sinus syndrome have bradyarrhythmia-related syncope or dizziness which may be associated with palpitations due to tachyarrhythmias.

Patients who present with symptomatic bradyarrhythmias due to chronic conduction system disease may require short-term support to maintain an adequate heart rate. If there is a history of dizziness or syncope associated with a ventricular rate of <40 b.p.m. (particularly if the escape rhythm is broad complex), or pauses of >3 seconds, then treatment is required. The options are:

- to commence an isoprenaline infusion (Appendix A) to increase the ventricular rate;
- to apply an external pacing system for temporary rate support;
- to insert a temporary pacing wire.

The complication rate for temporary pacing is high for inexperienced operators. The first two options are preferable in the absence of an appropriately skilled operator, and are discussed in more detail in Chapter 3. If temporary pacing is used, the femoral vein provides a good access site that minimizes the risk of access site complications and also reduces the amount of pacing lead manipulation required. If the patient has a rate of >40 b.p.m. with a narrow complex escape rhythm and no long pauses, it is appropriate to monitor the rhythm in a coronary care unit (CCU) environment, avoiding rhythm support initially. All patients with symptomatic chronic bradyarrhythmias should be considered for permanent pacing.

Key points

- Selecting the best treatment depends on the mechanism and effect of an arrhythmia.
- QRS duration is not a totally reliable guide to the site of origin of an arrhythmia.
- Antiarrhythmic drug therapy has many limitations (due to poor efficacy and side effects).
- AF is common – treatment depends on the duration of the arrhythmia and its haemodynamic effects. Atrial flutter is relatively uncommon, and is treated in a similar fashion to AF.
- The commonest cause of recurrent narrow complex tachycardia is AV nodal re-entry (which usually can be terminated by adenosine).

- Accessory pathways are not always associated with an abnormal resting ECG. The commonest associated arrhythmia is a regular narrow complex tachycardia with P waves visible between QRS complexes; AF is rare but can be dangerous.
- A broad complex tachycardia can be due to VT, bundle branch block or an accessory pathway. Most of these tachycardias are VT.
- Many bradyarrhythmias are well tolerated and emergency pacing should be avoided if possible.

Key references

Brugada P, Brugada J, Mont L, Smeets J, Andries EW. A new approach to the differential diagnosis of a regular tachycardia with a wide QRS complex. *Circulation* 1991; **83**: 1649–59.

Camm AJ, Garratt CJ. Adenosine and supraventricular tachycardia. *N Engl J Med* 1991; **325**: 1621–9.

DaCosta D, Brady WJ, Edhouse J. ABC of clinical electrocardiography. Bradycardias and atrioventricular conduction block. *BMJ* 2002; **324**: 535–8.

Dancy M, Ward D. Diagnosis of ventricular tachycardia: a clinical algorithm. *BMJ* 1989; **291**: 1036–8.

Edhouse J, Morris F. ABC of clinical electrocardiography. Broad complex tachycardia – Part I. *BMJ* 2002; **324**: 719–22.

Edhouse J, Morris F. ABC of clinical electrocardiography. Broad complex tachycardia – Part II. *BMJ* 2002; **324**: 776–9.

Esberger D, Jones S, Morris F. ABC of clinical electrocardiography: junctional tachycardias. *BMJ* 2002; **324**: 662–5.

Ganz LI, Friedman PL. Supraventricular tachycardia. *N Engl J Med* 1995; **332**: 162–73.

Goodacre S, Irons R. ABC of clinical electrocardiography: atrial arrhythmias. *BMJ* 2002; **324**: 594–7.

Julian DG. The amiodarone trials. *Eur Heart J* 1997; **18**: 1361–3.

Kowey PR, Marinchak RA, Rials SJ, Filart RA. Intravenous amiodarone. *J Am Coll Cardiol* 1997; **29**: 1190–8.

Levy S, Ricard P. Using the right drug: a treatment algorithm for regular supraventricular tachycardias. *Eur Heart J* 1997; **18**(Suppl C): C27–C32.

Murphy JJ. Problems with temporary cardiac pacing. *BMJ* 2001; **323**: 527.

Obel OA, Camm AJ. Supraventricular tachycardia: ECG and anatomy. *Eur Heart J* 1997; **18**(Suppl C): C2–C11.

Peters NS, Schilling RJ, Kanagaratnam P, Markides V. Atrial fibrillation: strategies to control, combat, and cure. *Lancet* 2002; **359**: 593–603.

Pye M, Camm AJ. Supraventricular tachycardia: a comprehensive review of the diagnosis and management of supraventricular tachycardia. *Hosp Update* 1996; **22**: 226–37.

Rankin AC, Cobbe SM. Broad-complex tachycardias. *Prescribers J* 1993; **33**: 138–46.

Roden DM. Risks and benefits of antiarrhythmic therapy. *N Engl J Med* 1994; **331**: 785–791.

Wellens HJJ. The value of the ECG in the diagnosis of supraventricular tachycardias. *Eur Heart J* 1996; **17**(Suppl C): 10–20.

Hypertensive emergencies

Background

Epidemiology

In a small proportion of patients with hypertension, an accelerated phase of the disease may develop. This presents clinically as a hypertensive emergency with marked elevation of blood pressure accompanied by end-organ damage. The incidence of hypertensive emergencies is declining due to widespread early treatment of less severe hypertension. Any hypertensive condition can develop into a crisis, although it is commoner in secondary forms of the disease such as with phaeochromocytoma and in renovascular hypertension. A hypertensive crisis is commonest in the young black male population. Prior to the introduction of effective anti-hypertensive therapy, less than 25 per cent of patients with malignant hypertension survived 1 year, with a 1 per cent 5-year survival. In the current era with renal dialysis support, 1- and 5-year survival is 90 per cent and 80 per cent, respectively. In severe hypertension, early death is usually due to stroke or acute renal failure. In the longer term, coronary artery disease becomes the commonest cause of death.

Hypertensive emergencies are most common in patients with long standing poorly controlled chronic hypertension. In these patients, chronic vascular changes provide a degree of protection to the end organs. In patients who develop an acute rise in blood pressure (for example, as a complication of acute renal failure or pregnancy) there are no chronic vascular adaptive changes to limit the adverse effects of the hypertension, and severe end-organ damage can occur at lower pressures.

Pathophysiology

The exact initiating step in a hypertensive crisis is not well understood. There is a cascade of physiological adaptation to a critical degree of hypertension, which occurs both systemically and locally in vascular beds. An increase in vasoreactivity occurs. The renin–angiotensin–aldosterone system is crucial in the development of this hyper-reactivity. Angiotensin II is a potent vasoconstrictor and also has direct cytotoxic effects on endothelium through activation of gene expression or pro-inflammatory cytokines such as interleukin-6 (IL-6) and the transcription factor, NF-Kβ. Inhibition of tissue angiotensin converting enzyme (ACE) can prevent malignant hypertension in transgenic mice. Systemically, there is activation of the sympathetic nervous system, the renin–angiotensin–aldosterone system and increased release of antidiuretic hormone. This leads to systemic vasoconstriction and an increase in circulating blood volume. Paradoxically, the baroreceptor response to this is overwhelmed with a further increase in circulating vasopressor hormones. Locally, free radical production and endothelin release is associated with further endothelial dysfunction, growth factor release and vascular smooth muscle cell proliferation diminishing local vascular autoregulation. Progressive endothelial dysfunction through pro-inflammatory cytokines with up-regulation of endothelial adhesion molecules (such as E- and P-selectin) promotes local inflammation. An increase in vascular permeability and activation of the coagulation cascade is the consequence of this, promoting further vasoconstriction. The end result of these adverse changes in neuroendocrine and vascular function is an acute rise in blood pressure, with diastolic pressures consistently exceeding 130 mmHg. The severe elevation in blood pressure leads to widespread necrosis in small arteries and arterioles. Thrombotic occlusion of these damaged vessels is common, leading to infarction in end organs. These damaged vessels also exhibit increased permeability leading to tissue oedema.

There are several important vascular beds which are at risk during a hypertensive emergency:

- **Cerebrovascular:** hypertensive encephalopathy is an acute medical emergency characterized by headache, irritability, an altered conscious level, seizures and coma. The acute diffuse neurological effects of malignant hypertension are reversed by prompt reduction in the blood pressure. Other potential complications of a hypertensive crisis are intracerebral or subarachnoid haemorrhage and a thrombotic infarction in an individual with predisposing atherosclerotic cerebrovascular disease.
- **Cardiovascular:** acute aortic dissection is the likeliest complication of a hypertensive crisis, particularly in patients with cystic medical necrosis of the thoracic aorta. Acute left ventricular failure (LVF) or an acute coronary syndrome may also occur.
- **Renal:** haematuria and progressive renal failure can occur.

Clinical evaluation

History

An accurate history of the duration and severity of any pre-existing hypertension must be established. It is equally important to establish the presence of end-organ damage, such as hypertensive renal disease and cerebrovascular disease. Symptoms of target organ injury may be present:

- anterior chest pain – myocardial ischaemia, acute aortic dissection;
- posterior chest pain – aortic dissection;
- dyspnoea – acute pulmonary oedema, chronic heart failure;
- altered consciousness/seizures – encephalopathy.

It is important to take a complete drug history to establish both any pre-existing therapy and the possibility of recent drug withdrawal. The recreational abuse of cocaine or other sympathomimetic drugs should be considered.

Physical examination

- Blood pressure measurement – in both arms, erect and supine
- Cardiovascular examination – presence of heart failure (raised jugular venous pressure (JVP), third heart sound, pulmonary crepitations)

- Neurological examination – conscious level, visual fields, focal pyramidal signs
- Fundoscopy – new haemorrhages, exudates and papilloedema indicate a hypertensive emergency

Initial investigations

- Biochemistry – urea, creatinine and electrolytes
- Haemotology – full blood count, including a blood film for evidence of haemolysis
- 12-lead ECG – to exclude/confirm ischaemia, to indicate left ventricular hypertrophy
- Chest radiograph
- Urinalysis – red blood cells, protein

Diagnostic features

Based on the history, physical examination and initial investigations, a hypertensive emergency can be diagnosed in the presence of:

- diastolic blood pressure greater than 140 mmHg;
- grade 3 or 4 hypertensive retinopathy;
- hypertensive encephalopathy;
- acute renal failure;
- microangiopathic haemolytic anaemia.

These patients require urgent blood pressure control to prevent early death.

Management

The treatment of a hypertensive crisis is based on consensus rather than on randomized controlled trials. The first principle of care is that a hypertensive emergency patient is managed in a high-dependency environment with withdrawal of any potential treatments that may be exacerbating the situation. This allows for accurate and continuous blood pressure monitoring with an arterial line. Treatment should be initiated by the intravenous route and titrated against the antihypertensive response. Combination therapy is preferred to achieve an additive effect and may be tailored towards any compromise in a particular end organ. In aortic dissection, a combination of intravenous beta-blockade (labetalol, which is a mixed alpha- and beta-blocker) given first followed by sodium nitroprusside is the preferred therapy. In the presence of myocardial ischaemia, intravenous glyceryl trinitrate with beta-blockade gives maximum anti-ischaemic effect with an antihypertensive effect. In hypertensive encephalopathy, centrally acting drugs should be avoided, and where cerebral infarction has occurred, rapid reductions in blood pressure should be avoided (blood pressure should be reduced gradually in patients with intracerebral and subarachnoid haemorrhage with diastolic pressures greater than 130 mmHg). The ideal time course for blood pressure reduction is to reduce mean arterial pressure by up to 25 per cent in the first 2 hours of treatment or to bring the diastolic pressure to between 100 and 110 mmHg within the same time period. In aortic dissection, a much greater reduction in diastolic pressure is required.

Specific drug therapy

Sodium nitroprusside

This short-acting arterial and venous dilator is first-line therapy for a hypertensive emergency. It has an immediate effect and its dose may be titrated against its efficacy. This will allow the simultaneous administration of oral antihypertensive agents, facilitating discontinuation of the nitroprusside infusion before the risk of thiocyanate toxicity. It is given in a dose of 0.25–10 μg/kg/min.

Labetalol

This mixed alpha- and beta-adrenergic blocker is the other mainstay of therapy in a hypertensive emergency. Although its beta-blocking effect is weaker than conventional beta-blockers, it can be given in bolus form at a dose of 20–80 mg in addition to an intravenous infusion of 2 mg/min.

ACE inhibition

These drugs are effective in lowering blood pressure within 15 minutes of an intravenous bolus such as enalapril (1.25–5 mg) with an effect lasting at least 4 hours. However, precipitous falls may occur in patients with hypovolaemia or significant renovascular disease. In accelerated hypertension, a pressure-induced natriuresis may occur, leading to the confounding physiological situation of hypovolaemia in the setting of hypertension.

Fenoldopam

This drug has been recently approved for use in hypertensive emergencies. It is a peripheral dopamine-1 receptor agonist, which peripherally vasodilates with an additional vasodilating effect on renal arteries. It is of quick onset (5 minutes) and is used at a dose of 0.1–0.6 µg/kg/min. In one study compared with sodium nitroprusside, fenoldopam improved renal dysfunction in severely hypertensive patients with renal impairment.

Glyceryl trinitrate (GTN)

Intravenous GTN (5–100 µg/min) is of particular use where significant coronary artery disease coexists with a hypertensive emergency. Although not a potent therapy for hypertension itself, the restoration of the imbalance between myocardial demand and supply through reduction in intramyocardial wall tension, preload reduction and improved collateral blood supply is of benefit, particularly when used in conjunction with beta-blockade. Like sodium nitroprusside, afterload reduction is of benefit in the presence of LVF.

Specific hypertensive emergencies

Hypertensive encephalopathy

There are both functional and structural processes which occur in the brain when there is an acute sustained increase in systemic blood pressure. The functional response to an excessive perfusion pressure is cerebral arteriolar vasodilatation (rather than vasoconstriction as expected) and a loss of microcirculatory autoregulation, leading to the leakage of fluid into the perivascular space and cerebral oedema. With acute endothelial injury, the structural changes in the arterioles lead to an increase in vascular permeability independent of the renin–angiotensin–aldosterone system. This leads to disruption of the blood–brain barrier, cerebral oedema, and microhaemorrhage. The normal range over which vital organs such as the brain and the heart autoregulate blood flow in the face of varying perfusion pressure is between 60 and 120 mmHg.

In patients with pre-existing hypertension, this autoregulatory range is increased to between 110 and 180 mmHg through an increase in the intimal area of the larger resistive vessels (pre-arterioles) that deliver perfusion to the smaller resistive vessels (arterioles). These former vessels are influenced by the perfusion pressure and cerebral blood flow, and by myogenic tone. Conversely, in patients with no previous hypertension, signs of encephalopathy can occur at a pressure as low as 160/100 mmHg. Thus, the clinical response is largely dependent on whether the patient develops the hypertensive crisis in the context of a previously normal blood pressure.

Hypertensive encephalopathy is characterized by the acute onset of lethargy, confusion, headache, visual disturbance and focal or generalized seizures. If untreated, coma, cerebral haemorrhage and death may ensue. Intracerebral haemorrhage is particularly likely in thrombotic thrombocytopenic purpura and in pre-eclampsia where haemolysis occurs with acute liver injury and thrombocytopenia occurs. Magnetic resonance imaging with T_2-weighting may confirm a posterior leucoencephalopathy affecting predominantly the white matter of the parieto-occipital regions (largely bilateral). The cerebellum and brainstem may also be affected, and occasionally the cerebral cortex. The posterior cerebral predilection occurs through a reduction in sympathetic innervation accompanying the basilar artery and its branches.

Hypertensive encephalopathy is reversible, leading to the specific term hypertensive reversible posterior leucoencephalopathy syndrome (PLS). It has been described in both children and adults and may also occur in non-hypertensive situations such as through drug toxicity [cyclosporin and tacrolimus (often an acute cause of hypertension), cisplatin and interferon-α therapy], acquired immunodeficiency syndrome (AIDS), thrombotic thrombocytopenic purpura and after blood tranfusion.

Although the aim of treatment is to bring the diastolic pressure down to around 100 mmHg within the first hour, it is important to be aware that patients with pre-existing hypertension and elderly patients are at particular risk of a watershed infarct with aggressive blood pressure reduction. In patients with seizure activity, anticonvulsant therapy using intravenous phenytoin or benzodiazepines should be given additionally.

Phaeochromocytoma

Phaeochromocytoma arise from sympathetic ganglia derived from the primitive neural crest with 90 per cent arising from the adrenal medulla,

10 per cent bilateral and 10 per cent malignant rather than benign. They account for 0.1 per cent of hypertensive patients. These 'tumours', which are essentially extreme nodular hyperplasia, may occur as part of the familial multiple endocrine neoplasia (MEN-2) syndrome. They create extreme fluctuations in systemic blood pressure with associated symptoms, although the hypertension becomes persistent in half of patients. With adrenaline as the predominant catecholamine secreted (mainly from adrenal medullary tumours), symptoms of an increased cardiac output with systolic hypertension, sinus tachycardia, sweating, flushing and apprehension occur. When noradrenaline is the predominant hormone (adrenal and most extra-adrenal tumours), there is an increased peripheral vasoconstriction with diastolic as well as systolic hypertension with less tachycardia or palpitations. If the hypertension is paroxysmal, it often occurs in response to anaesthesia, parturition, or pharmacological stress from histamine, caffeine, beta-blockade or glucocorticoids.

A direct relationship between high levels of catecholamines and myocardial injury exists with the potential for myocarditis and acute left ventricular failure. Diagnosis is made simply through a 24-hour urine collection for urinary metanephrines. To improve the specificity of this test, patients should have monoamine oxidase inhibitors and mixed alpha- and beta-blockers (labetalol, carvedilol) discontinued beforehand. The tumour may be localized by CT scanning with the occasional need for radioisotope localization with MIBG. Where possible, phaeochromocytoma should be resected with careful pre- and peri-operative alpha-adrenoceptor blockade (with intravenous phentolamine at 5–10 µg/min) to diminish vasoconstriction and allow intravascular volume expansion.

Hypertensive emergencies in pregnancy

The term gestational hypertension now covers the clinical syndrome of new-onset hypertension in the last trimester of pregnancy. The term eclampsia refers to the development of convulsions as a conseqeunce of acute gestational hypertension (pre-eclampsia). Gestational hypertension is more common in primigravida and in situations where there are racial differences between parents. Predisposing variables include older maternal age, black race, multiple gestations, concomitant renal disease and pre-existing hypertension. It is a self-limiting condition with resolution after delivery and is characterized by sudden weight gain and oedema, retinal oedema, proteinuria and an increased plasma urate.

An increased susceptibility to hypertensive encephalopathy exists due to the lack of previous hypertension in the mother and thus a breakthrough of increased cerebral blood flow from autoregulation which may lead to cerebral oedema and seizures.

The unifying cause of gestational hypertension is a reduction in uteroplacental perfusion and subsequent decrease in prostaglandin production and prostacyclin in particular. Although there was a vogue for the use of low dose aspirin (<100 mg) to inhibit thromboxane production and prevent the development of gestational hypertension, this approach remains controversial given the increased risk of excessive bleeding during delivery.

The traditional approach to management has been bed rest and drug therapy with methyldopa, given its long-term safety profile, with the use of intravenous hydralazine around the time of delivery. However, beta-blockers, the alpha-blocker prazosin, labetalol and nifedipine have also been used with success. Furthermore, intravenous magnesium should be given in pre-eclampsia to prevent the development of seizure activity. A concern with the use of drugs, particularly beta-blockade, in mild gestational hypertension is the risk of intrauterine growth retardation with little effect on blood pressure control compared to simple bed rest alone. Should eclampsia supervene, patients should receive intravenous diazepam immediately to control seizure activity. Haemodynamic monitoring is recommended given the need to optimize intravascular volume status in the presence of oliguria (fluid challenge) or increased loading conditions (vasodilatation).

Hypertensive emergencies in critical illness

In critical illness, there are many factors which can increase catecholamine production and increase vasoconstriction leading to an acute elevation of blood pressure. Post-anaesthetic sympathomimetic stimulation, fluid overload and hypothermia are common causes of hypertension in critically ill patients. Hypertensive crises may occur in up to 5 per cent of intensive care unit patients. These may be treated by non-pharmacological means in the first instance over a period of 15 minutes although these measures are likely to be effective in a minority of patients. Such treatments include the relief of anxiety, pain, or both; correction of hypoxia; patient instrumentation adjustment such as of mechanical ventilation and nasogastric tubes or urinary catheters; and correction of circulating blood volume and electrolyte imbalance.

Key points

- In about 1 per cent of patients with hypertension, an accelerated phase may occur as part of the progression of the disease and is commonest in the young black male population. It is commoner in secondary forms of the disease such as with phaeochromocytoma and in renovascular hypertension.
- Prior to established antihypertensive therapy, less than 25 per cent of patients with malignant hypertension survived 1 year, with a 1 per cent 5-year survival. In the current era with renal dialysis support, 1- and 5-year survival is 90 per cent and 80 per cent, respectively. Early death tends to occur due to stroke or acute renal failure.
- Malignant hypertension is the clinical syndrome where a sudden increased systemic blood pressure is likely to result in acute end-organ injury. The likelihood of this may vary according to pre-existing levels and to the rate of the acute rise, although it is accepted that a persistent diastolic blood pressure of greater than 130 mmHg is likely to result in vascular injury.
- The clinical features of a hypertensive crisis comprise a diastolic blood pressure greater than 130–140 mmHg, hypertensive retinopathy, hypertensive encephalopathy, acute renal failure, and microangiopathic haemolytic anaemia.
- Hypertensive encephalopathy is an acute medical emergency characterized by headache, irritability and an altered conscious level. Other potential complications of a hypertensive crisis are an intracerebral or subarachnoid haemorrhage and a thrombotic infarction in an individual with predisposing atherosclerotic cerebrovascular disease.
- Acute aortic dissection is the likeliest cardiac complication of a hypertensive crisis, particularly in patients with cystic medial necrosis of the thoracic aorta. Acute left ventricular failure or an acute coronary syndrome may also occur.
- A hypertensive emergency patient should be managed in a high-dependency environment with withdrawal of any potential treatments which may be exacerbating the situation. Treatment should be initiated by the intravenous route and titrated against antihypertensive response. Combination drug therapy is preferred to achieve an additive effect and may be tailored towards any compromise in a particular end-organ.
- Sodium nitroprusside (a short-acting arterial and venous dilator) is first-line therapy for a hypertensive emergency. It has an

immediate effect and its dose may be titrated against its efficacy and allow the administration of oral antihypertensive agents to allow discontinuation before the risk of thiocyanate toxicity.

- Labetalol (a mixed alpha- and beta-adrenergic blocker) is the other mainstay of therapy in a hypertensive emergency given as bolus and intravenous infusion.

- Gestational hypertension is the clinical syndrome of new-onset hypertension in the last trimester of pregnancy. It is more common in primigravida and in situations where there are racial differences between parents. Predisposing variables include older maternal age, black race, multiple gestations, concomitant renal disease and pre-existing hypertension. It is self-limiting with resolution after delivery and is characterized by sudden weight gain and oedema, retinal oedema, and proteinuria.

Key references

Bennett NM, Shea S. Hypertensive emergency: case criteria, socio-demographic profile, and previous case of 100 cases. *Am J Public Health* 1988; **78**: 636–42.

Calhoun DA, Oparil S. Treatment of hypertensive crisis. *N Engl J Med* 1990; **323**: 1177–83.

Cumming AM, Davies DL. Intravenous labetalol in hypertensive emergency. *Lancet* 1979; **i**: 929–30.

Finnerty FA. Hypertensive encephalopathy. *Am J Med* 1972; **52**: 672–8.

Koch-Weser J. Hypertensive emergencies. *N Engl J Med* 1974; **290**: 211–14.

Lucas MJ, Levenko KJ, Cunningham FG. A comparison of magnesium sulphate with phenytoin for the prevention of eclampsia. *N Engl J Med* 1995; **333**: 201–5.

Montgomery HE, Kiernan LA, Whotworth CE *et al.* Inhibition of tissue angiotensin converting enzyme activity prevents malignant hypertension in TGR(mREN2)27. *J Hypertens* 1998; **16**: 635–43.

Schiff E, Peleg E, Goldenberg M *et al.* The use of aspirin to reduce pregnancy-induced hypertension and lower the ratio of thromboxane A_2 to prostacyclin in relatively high-risk pregnancies. *N Engl J Med* 1989; **321**: 351–7.

Shusterman NH, Elliott WJ, White WB. Fenoldopam, but not nitroprusside improves renal function in severely hypertensive patients with impaired renal function. *Am J Med* 1993; **95**: 161–8.

Vaughan CJ, Delanty N. Hypertensive emergencies. *Lancet* 2000; **356**: 411–17.

Wilson DJ, Wallin JD, Vlachakis ND. Intravenous labetalol in the treatment of severe hypertension and hypertensive emergencies. *Am J Med* 1983; **75**(Suppl): 95–102.

Aortic emergencies

Background

Epidemiology

Dissection of the thoracic aorta is one the most dramatic acute medical emergencies with serious adverse consequences if not diagnosed and treated promptly and appropriately. It has been estimated that there are between 10 and 20 cases per million population per year, most commonly occurring in men aged between 50 and 70 years, and more often in the black population. On average, left untreated, 50 per cent of patients die within 48 hours (estimated at a 1 per cent mortality per hour from presentation) with 70 per cent dead at 1 week and 90 per cent dead at 3 months.

Definition and classification

Thoracic aortic dissection has been classified on anatomical grounds with regard to the origin and extent of the dissection and this has major implications in the treatment of the condition. The thoracic aorta is most likely to dissect at either the ascending aorta or in the descending aorta just below the left subclavian artery. The original classification by DeBakey described three different types:

- type I – dissection in the ascending thoracic aorta extending round the arch into the descending aorta and into the abdomen;
- type II – dissection in the ascending thoracic aorta only with no distal extension past the innominate artery;
- type III – dissection in the descending thoracic aorta distal to the left subclavian artery. Retrograde extension may occasionally occur back into the thoracic aortic arch and ascending aorta. In one follow-up study of aortic dissection, this subtype was subclassified into IIIa (limited to thoracic aorta) and IIIb (extension into the abdominal aorta).

The natural history of types I and II are similar and have led to the simpler Stanford classification of:

- type A, where dissection arises in the ascending aorta irrespective of its extension; and
- type B, equivalent to DeBakey type III, but excluding dissections with retrograde extension into the arch.

Rarely, a three-channelled dissection can occur where dissection occurs twice in the natural history of an individual patient (A + B or B + B, rarely A + A) in whom there is usually a high incidence of Marfan's syndrome.

Pathophysiology

Acute aortic dissection is strongly associated with systemic hypertension (due to a sustained high intraluminal pressure) and with advancing age. Cystic medial degeneration in the aortic wall is an intrinsic feature of several connective tissue disorders which are associated with dissection such as Marfan's syndrome, Ehlers–Danlos syndrome, and occasionally, giant cell aortitis. These patients are at particular risk of dissection, often at a young age. There is an increased association with a bicuspid aortic valve and coarctation of the aorta, and thus with Turner's syndrome as well as Noonan's syndrome. Dissection can be seen in the last trimester of pregnancy and at the site of a previous surgical aortotomy. The presence of atherosclerosis *per se* does not predispose to thoracic aortic dissection but is associated with saccular aneurysmal dilatation. However, rupture of an intimal plaque in older patients remains a mechanism for dissection.

Degeneration of the collagen and elastin matrix within the aortic medial layer is the chief predisposition in most cases of aortic dissection.

The direct mechanism of dissection is unclear as the same pathological process may occur either through intimal rupture with secondary dissection into media, or primary medial haemorrhage with local
disruption of the intima. An intimal tear is not absolute in the pathology
of the dissecting process as extensive intramural haematoma may occur
without a discernible intimal disruption through rupture of the vasa
vasorum within the aortic media, culminating in the formation of a
haematoma, which may remain confined within the media or propagate, with eventual rupture through the intimal layer. Penetrating
ulcers, which are part of the same pathological process, are typically
found in the descending thoracic or abdominal aorta. The penetrating
atherosclerotic ulcer is characterized by focal contrast enhancement or
filling defects beyond the confines of the aorta with persisting luminal
communication. Although there are limited data regarding natural history, mortality and morbidity following intramural haematoma and
aortic ulceration are similar to those of classical dissection and it now
appears that they may represent a precursor of dissection rather than a
separate entity.

The formation of a tear in the aortic intima allows penetration of blood
into the diseased medial layer at arterial pressure, separating the laminar
plane of the media and dissecting the aortic wall. This dissection process
may extend a variable distance, usually in an antegrade direction, but
sometimes retrogradely from the site of the intimal tear. The blood-filled
space between the dissected layers of the aortic wall becomes the false
lumen. Shear forces may cause further tears in the intimal flap, producing exit sites or additional entry sites for blood flow in the false lumen.
Eventually, distension of the false lumen may cause the intimal flap to
bow into the true lumen, thereby narrowing its calibre and distorting its
shape. The circulation of any major arterial vessel can be compromised
by the dissection process, leading to ischaemia. The aortic valve may be
disrupted, leading to aortic regurgitation. The dissecting process may
rupture through the adventitia at any point, commonly into the pericardial space or left pleural cavity.

Clinical manifestations of aortic dissection

Aortic dissection can mimic several different intrathoracic pathologies
in the evolution of the symptoms and signs. The common clinical features are:

- severe chest pain – this is the commonest symptom of dissection.
  It is as severe at its outset as at any other time and is unremitting.

It is often described as 'tearing' in nature. The pain tends to migrate as the dissecting haematoma extends. Anterior chest pain is common with proximal dissection whereas interscapular pain is common in descending aortic dissection and may be in both areas where a type I dissection has occurred. Pain may be noted in the neck and jaw where the ascending aorta or arch is involved.

- vasovagal symptoms – acute diaphoresis with sweating, apprehension and syncope are common.
- altered blood pressure – many patients are hypertensive at presentation. Conversely, hypotension may occur through cardiac tamponade, aortic rupture, or dissection in the head and neck vessels, leading to a reduced perfusion pressure in the brachial artery (pseudohypotension) and thus pulse deficits. Pulse deficits are commonly associated with proximal dissection in the brachiocephalic vessels or less commonly through involvement of the left subclavian artery from a distal dissection. The loss of a pulse may occur either through an occlusive intimal flap at a vascular orifice or through direct compression of an artery lumen.
- aortic valve regurgitation – this occurs either through a circumferential tear opening up the annulus and reducing coaptation, distortion of the valve apparatus through asymmetric dissection, or through direct disruption of the annular support, leading to a flail leaflet. It occurs in up to two-thirds of proximal dissection. If severe, acute left ventricular failure may ensue from acute aortic insufficiency.
- right coronary artery dissection – leading to an acute inferior myocardial infarction (MI).
- acute neurological deficits – ischaemic stroke, altered consciousness and paraparesis due to spinal cord ischaemia are most common with proximal dissections.
- mediastinal complications – these occur through the expansion of the dissection with compression of the superior cervical sympathetic ganglion (Horner's syndrome), compression of the left recurrent laryngeal nerve (hoarseness), superior vena caval compression, and tracheal compression.
- pleural effusion – usually occurs on the left and is due to either rupture into the pleural space or an inflammatory exudate.
- acute rupture – in addition to the pericardial space and pleural and intra-abdominal cavities, haemorrhage into the lung, oesophagus or rupture into right atrium may, rarely, occur.
- visceral infarction – mesenteric and renal infarction may occur in dissections spreading into the abdominal aorta.

Diagnosis of aortic dissection

Sudden onset of non-ischaemic, non-pleuritic chest pain is common in several acute cardiovascular disorders with classical aortic dissection (and its variants intramural haematoma and penetrating atherosclerotic ulcer) the commonest diagnosis. To make this diagnosis, it is important to exclude thoracic aortic aneurysm, aortic rupture, acute pulmonary embolism (PE) and complications following cardiothoracic surgery; this is most accurately done with spiral computed tomography (CT), although transoesophageal echocardiogram (TOE) is the preferred diagnostic method in many places as it is portable, rapidly performed, sensitive and specific, and does not require the use of contrast agents. The important diagnostic investigational features are:

- 12-lead electrocardiogram (ECG). The ECG may be within normal limits in the absence of coronary artery dissection. In the presence of pre-existing hypertension, left ventricular hypertrophy may be present.
- chest radiology. A widened mediastinum is a classical finding in thoracic aortic dissection. There may be an additional local bulge at the site of dissection. The presence of a left pleural effusion and tracheal deviation are often seen. Separation of calcification in the aortic arch from the apparent adventitial border is a powerful sign of dissection. However, extensive dissection can occur in the presence of a normal chest x-ray.
- echocardiography. Transthoracic echocardiography will detect a proximal dissection where a dilated aortic root is present but is limited in any further delineation of a dissection. TOE allows visualization of the aortic root, proximal ascending aorta and descending aorta. With colour-flow doppler, entry and exit sites between true and false lumen may be identified. With intramural haematoma, an echolucent crescentic region should be seen over a length of the aorta. Occasionally, the haematoma is circumferential and can be difficult to differentiate from common atherosclerotic thickening. An important disadvantage is its limited ability to visualize the distal ascending aorta and proximal arch due to interposition of the trachea and left main bronchus. Furthermore, it is unable to image beyond the distal thoracic descending aorta and thus cannot assess the iliac vessels – an important limitation where endoluminal repair is being considered.
- computed tomography (CT). CT with an intravenous contrast injection to enhance the intraluminal phase is, in general, the

investigation of choice in most acute medical environments, given a reported sensitivity and specificity approaching 100 per cent. With the presence of a membrane (intimal flap), the false and true lumina can be identified. The false lumen is usually the larger of the two; CT scanning has the disadvantage that it is unable to provide haemodynamic information, relies upon the use of nephrotoxic contrast agents and may be unable to depict branch-vessel involvement. Spiral CT (which involves shorter screening times and allows two- and three-dimensional reconstruction) is useful in the follow-up of dissection by allowing assessment of early and late changes after surgery or medical treatment such as postoperative complications of type A dissection, healing of intramural haematoma, progression of intramural haematoma, and aneurysms of the true and false lumina. Monitoring of compromised abdominal branch vessels may be performed. CT angiography can demonstrate complex spatial relationships, mural abnormalities and extraluminal pathologies.

- magnetic resonance imaging (MRI). MRI may used as an alternative imaging technology without the need for contrast and with enhanced resolution. MRI gives an improved anatomic delineation of the aorta and can provide high quality images in several planes, including a left anterior oblique view that displays the entire thoracic aorta. Furthermore, MRI is superior to conventional CT in differentiating acute intramural haematoma from atherosclerotic plaque and chronic intraluminal thrombus.

- aortic angiography. With the improvements made in echocardiographic and tomographic imaging, the vogue for invasive confirmation has diminished. The intention of angiography is to identify the site of origin and to delineate the extent of the dissection. The procedure carries with it a significant mortality and should largely be reserved for cases where the diagnosis is uncertain. It is of no help in the diagnosis of intramural haematoma.

Because symptoms may mimic more common disorders such as MI and acute aortic regurgitation and because characteristic physical findings such as a pulse deficit may be absent, dissection may be difficult to diagnose. It should be suspected in any patient presenting with chest or interscapular pain and diaphoresis. The International Registry of Acute Aortic Dissection (IRAD), established in 1996, has reported trends in the management and outcome of the condition. Classical clinical findings were infrequent and the initial ECG and chest x-ray were often normal. CT was the initial imaging modality in 61 per cent.

Treatment of aortic dissection

Immediate therapy

All patients in whom a thoracic aortic dissection is suspected should be monitored and treated in a high dependency environment for haemodynamic and cardiac rhythm monitoring and for central venous access. Patients should be cross-matched for the eventuality of either dissection or rupture and early surgery. The two initial goals of therapy are:

- to alleviate pain with intravenous opiate analgesia, and
- to reduce systolic pressure to a range of 100–120 mmHg, equivalent to a mean arterial pressure of 60–75 mmHg, and sufficient to maintain vital organ perfusion.

Third, the velocity of left ventricular ejection (the dP/dt) should be reduced by beta-blockade independently of systemic blood pressure lowering.

Blood pressure lowering is achieved by an infusion of intravenous sodium nitroprusside up to a maximum dose of 400 μg/min (5 μg/kg/min). The infusion should not be given for more than 48 hours due to the risk of cyanide toxicity. Frequent blood gases should be taken for acid–base status (a metabolic acidosis tends to develop with cyanide toxicity). Concomitant infusion of vitamin B_{12} (hydroxocobalamin) reduces plasma cyanide levels through the formation of cyanocobalamin. Sodium nitroprusside reduces the blood pressure but may actually increase the dP/dt through afterload reduction. Intravenous beta-blockade is used to reduce dP/dt. The most popular agent used is labetalol, which is a non-selective beta-blocker and alpha-blocker. It can be given either as bolus doses of 5–20 mg up to a total of 300 mg or may be given as an infusion (see Appendix A).

Definitive treatment

The accepted paradigm in dissection management is that surgical treatment is superior to medical treatment in the management of type A dissection, whereas medical therapy is superior in uncomplicated type B dissection (see Box 6.1). This comes about through surgery preventing progression of dissection and potentially fatal consequences. Patients with distal dissection tend to be older with atherosclerotic vascular disease, often with a reduced cardiac reserve, and tend to tolerate surgery

Box 6.1 Indications for specific treatment of aortic dissection

Surgery
- Acute type A dissection
- Acute type B dissection with complications
  - compromised perfusion to vital organs
  - rupture/ threatened rupture
  - retrograde dissection to ascending aorta/aortic valve regurgitation
  - Marfan's syndrome
  - inability or control pain
  - saccular aneurysm formation
- Chronic dissection with complications
  - progressive aortic dilatation (>50 mm maximum diameter)
  - persistent false lumen in communication with the true lumen
  - persistent pain

Medical therapy
- Uncomplicated type B dissection
- Uncomplicated arch dissection
- Stable chronic dissection

less well, favouring medical therapy. The attrition rate in patients with proximal dissection treated surgically occurs through complications having already occurred or through the friability of the aortic wall at surgery.

Surgery

Current practice dictates that the proximal dissection should be repaired early to prevent extension and rupture, and to operate on distal dissections extending proximally using cardiopulmonary bypass. The intimal tear is excised and the origin of the false lumen excluded by proximal and distal suturing of the edges of aorta. A prosthetic Dacron graft may be needed to approximate the ends of the aorta. An alternative technique is to wrap the aorta with Dacron. Where the aortic valve is involved, the false channel is decompressed by the surgery described above, but may still require to be replaced. Where the aorta is very friable, the whole ascending aorta and valve may be replaced using a composite graft containing a mechanical prosthesis with resuturing of the coronary arteries to the conduit. Preservation of the native aortic valve, which avoids the complications associated with a prosthetic valve, usually requires approximation of the two layers of dissected aortic wall and resuspension of the commissures with pledgeted sutures. However, prosthetic valve replacement is frequently advisable in the setting of pre-existent valve disease or in Marfan's syndrome to reduce the likelihood of reoperation.

Several different surgical adaptations have occurred to improve outcome. A Dacron sleeve may be used to bypass the dissection (usually in the descending aorta) with ligation of aorta at the dissection's proximal extension, thus creating reverse flow in the distal aorta. Others have advocated the use of sponge insertion into the false lumen to promote organization of thrombus or the innovative use of a gelatin–resorcinol–formaldehyde (GRF) glue to adhere the proximal layers of the dissection without the need for a prosthetic graft. In a review of experience of aortic valve preservation and aortic root reconstruction in type A dissection, 121 patients with this operation (with one or more sinuses of Valsalva reconstructed) from a total of 246 were reported. A total of 25 per cent of patients were in cardiogenic shock at operation. Additional reinforcement of the aortic root was achieved with Teflon felt, GRF glue, or fibrinous glue. An operative mortality of 21.5 per cent occurred with a 53 per cent survival at 10 years (with a freedom from aortic root reoperation of 69 per cent at 10 years). Risk factors for reoperation were the use of fibrinous glue and an aortic annulus of greater than 27 mm.

Surgical fenestration has been used as a means of decompressing an occlusive false lumen in the descending aorta in patients with visceral or limb ischaemia. A retrospective review of this procedure performed between 1979 and 1999 at the Mayo Clinic has been reported in 14 patients with acute (7) and chronic (7) dissection. Three were type A and 11 were type B. Fenestration may be performed alongside ascending aortic surgery and additional abdominal aortic grafting. It can also be done percutaneously and is usually done in the pararenal or infrarenal area. In all 10 patients with malperfusion, flow was restored. However, operative mortality for emergency fenestration was 43 per cent, but there were no postoperative deaths in the elective fenestration group with no late recurrence of malperfusion or aneurysm formation.

Percutaneous interventional treatment

In type B dissection, the persistence of a false lumen has an adverse effect of clinical outcome (higher rates of reoperation and mortality) where an active communication persists between true and false lumina, compared to where there is thrombosis of the false lumen. The deployment of balloon-expandable or self-expanding endoluminal stents may be performed to re-establish flow into branch vessels compromised by dissection into the origin of the vessel. If a branch vessel is compromised by pressure from the false lumen over the origin of the vessel, a fenestration procedure may be undertaken to decompress the false lumen.

Similarly, endoluminal exclusion with a stent graft prosthesis [consisting of circumferential nitinol stent springs arranged as a tube and covered with a Dacron or polytetrafluoroethylene (PTFE) graft exterior] placed over the false lumen entry site will decompress the false lumen, causing the flap to oppose the aortic wall and relieve branch vessel compromise. The advantage of endoluminal exclusion in acute dissection is that it combines closure of the false lumen and prevents subsequent dilatation with relief of branch vessel obstruction. Stent grafts are sized by measurement from pre-procedure imaging. They require a proximal neck of ideally 20 mm of 'normal aorta' above the false lumen origin to ensure secure deployment against the aortic wall. The potential for ischaemia through occlusion of the left arm vascular supply may be predicted by preliminary occlusive balloon inflation for 20 minutes in the left subclavian artery to assess the integrity of the collateral circulation, perhaps using a partially covered graft if necessary. The position of the undeployed graft may be obtained using aortography, intravascular ultrasound or TOE. The distal neck may be normal supracoeliac aorta or biluminal descending thoracic aorta. In the absence of a distal neck, the shortest graft that effectively covers the entry site is used.

TOE may be used in combination with fluoroscopy and angiography in monitoring the outcome of stent-graft placement. It allows accurate positioning of the stent-graft away from significant atheroma and calcification and colour doppler assessment indentifies peri-graft leak more often than angiography, allowing additional balloon dilatation or a second stent-graft. Stent-grafts can be used not only for type B dissections but also for thoracic and thoraco-abdominal aneurysms, and for post-traumatic aortic dissections.

As described above, the fenestration technique may be employed using an endovascular approach (usually as a bridge to definitive endoluminal repair) using a needle to pass a wire, then balloon dilatation of the puncture site. In one series of 40 patients with peripheral ischaemic complications of aortic dissection (10 type A, 30 type B), 14 were treated with a stent in the true or false lumen combined with fenestration of the intimal flap, 24 had stenting alone, and 2 had fenestration alone. Successful revascularization was achieved in 37 patients (93 per cent) with a 30-day mortality rate of 25 per cent, largely related to pre-existent irreversible ischaemia. In cases where endoluminal repair or fenestration is considered, digital subtraction angiography, or magnetic resonance angiography is an essential prelude to allow assessment of the access arteries (usually the iliacs), measurement of the aorta to permit selection of the correct device length and diameter, confirmation of branch vessel involvement and biluminal manometry prior to fenestration.

Penetrating atherosclerotic ulceration and intramural aortic haematoma

These pathological variations of aortic dissection are radiologically distinct from classical dissection. In penetrating atherosclerotic ulcers (PAU), no intimal flap is demonstrable with a crater visible, extending into the aortic wall and associated with haematoma within the media of the aortic wall. An intramural haematoma (IMH) is present where significant thickening or enhancement of the aortic wall is seen in the absence of a flap or dissection. In one recent review of 214 cases presenting as aortic dissection, 36 cases were re-defined as either PAU or IMH, thus accounting for one-eighth of cases of 'dissection'.

The clinical course of these two variants may differ from dissection. Patients with PAU/IMH are older than type A dissection (74 years vs 56 years, $P < 0.001$) and tend to be older than type B dissections, and thus are commonest between the seventh and ninth decades. Patients with PAU/IMH are almost always hypertensive (94 per cent). PAU and IMH are most common in the descending aorta (90 per cent and 71 per cent, respectively). The presentation with anterior or posterior chest pain is similar to that of classical dissection. However, PAU/IMH do not cause arterial vessel compromise and thus distal limb ischaemia or visceral compromise, and tend to be focal without propagation. Penetrating ulcers are uniformly associated with severe aortic atherosclerosis, usually with calcification, in contrast to classical dissection, which has little association with atherosclerosis. PAU and IMH tend to occur in more dilated aortae (62 mm and 55 mm vs 52 mm, $P < 0.05$) and have an association with abdominal aortic aneurysms (42 per cent of PAU and 29 per cent of IMH).

It is thought likely that the radial level in the wall at which an intramural haematoma occurs determines whether an acute dissection or haematoma develops. It may be that if blood collects closer to the adventitia, there is less likelihood of intimal rupture. This would also explain a higher external rupture rate with IMH, which tends to run a more malignant course than typical descending aortic dissection.

The treatment of IMH is similar to that of classical aortic dissection. In one recent retrospective review, 51 patients (36 male) with IMH and a mean age of 67 years were reported. The ascending aorta or arch was involved in 18 patients (group I) with the descending aorta in 33 patients (group II). Intimal disruption was noted in 55 per cent of the former and in 39 per cent of the latter group. In the group I patients, the 2-year survival rate was 94 per cent with 75 per cent of this group undergoing surgery. Immediate surgery was performed for cardiac tamponade, superimposed dissection, and persistent pain with an aortic arch aneurysm. Early elective operations were done for an enlarging ulcer and for aneurysmal dilatation. In group II, 9/33 (27 per cent) patients underwent surgery mainly for intimal disruption. An enlarging ulcer necessitated crossover to surgery in four patients. The 5-year survival in this group was 63 per cent with 66 per cent remaining free from surgery. It is imperative that patients with penetrating ulcers treated medically are followed up because of the potential to enlargement, particularly in the first month.

An attempt to identify those patients with type A IMH who are likely to require surgery has been done with serial CT scanning of 22 patients. The aortic diameter and wall thickness were measured at three different levels on admission and at follow-up (at a mean of 37 days). In one group ($n = 10$), progression of maximal aortic wall thickness or rupture occurred compared to the remaining patients who regressed. The maximal initial aortic wall diameter was greater (55 ± 6 vs 47 ± 3 mm, $P = 0.001$) in the group who progressed. A cut-off value of 50 mm gave a positive predictive accuracy of 83 per cent for progression of type A IMH. In another group of 21 patients with IMH, patients with the type A form had a prognosis similar to that of type A dissections. In the remaining patients with aortic arch or type B IMH, a more benign course was reported.

Clinical outcome in aortic dissection

From the International Registry of Acute Aortic Dissection, overall in-hospital mortality was 27.4 per cent:

- type A
  – surgical management 26 per cent
  – medical management 58 per cent
- type B
  – surgical management 31 per cent
  – medical management 11 per cent.

These high mortality rates have been confirmed in several other large series. Moreover, for acute disease complicated by end-organ ischaemia, surgical mortality exceeds 50 per cent, with a substantial risk (7–36 per cent) of paraplegia (or paresis), dependent upon the extent of aortic dissection and the duration of cross-clamping, amongst those who survive. Chronic aortic dissection (presentation up to 2 weeks after the onset of symptoms) has a higher in-hospital survival of around 90 per cent whether they are treated medically or surgically, largely through self-selection due to the lack of acute complications in the initial phase of dissection.

The initial success of surgical or medical therapy is usually sustained at long-term follow-up with typical 5-year survival rates of 75–82 per cent. There appear to be no major differences amongst groups according to the site of dissection, mode of presentation, or treatment. A number of clinical factors have been linked with poor prognosis in addition to the anatomy of the dissection. Acute complications at the time of acute presentation, such as a cerebrovascular accident, MI, severe aortic regurgitation, renal failure, mesenteric infarction and lower limb ischaemia, in addition to aneurysmal dilatation of the dissected aorta and increasing age, predict an adverse outcome.

The incidence of aneurysm formation at a site remote from the original surgical repair is 17–25 per cent with the majority appearing within 2 years. Many arise from dilatation of the residual false lumen in the distal unresected aortic segments and are prone to rupture owing to their relatively thin outer wall. To identify such a development, careful long-term follow-up with serial aortic imaging, usually using MRI, is recommended. Patients are at highest risk during the first 2 years and should be assessed every 3–6 months during this period. Thereafter, they should be re-evaluated every 6–12 months according to their perceived individual risk.

New developments

Trials in percutaneous stent-grafting

The use of percutaneous technology to treat type B dissections is the major growth area in aortic dissection management. Using covered stent-grafts, Dake et al. reported outcome in 19 patients with acute type B dissection (four with retrograde extension into the proximal aorta). One-third of patients had branch vessel compromise – stent-grafts were deployed successfully across the primary entry tear in all patients with complete thrombosis of the false lumen in 15 (the remainder had partial thrombosis) with an early mortality of 16 per cent. There were no late deaths, nor instances of aneurysm or aortic rupture during subsequent follow-up to 1 year. In another randomized trial, Nienaber et al. (1999) compared the outcome in 12 patients with subacute or chronic type B dissection treated using a self-expanding nitinol tubular stent-graft coated with Dacron with 12 matched surgical controls. Stent-graft placement resulted in no morbidity or mortality, whereas surgery was associated with a 33 per cent mortality and 42 per cent serious adverse events. Follow-up MRI at 3 months confirmed thrombosis of the false lumen in all 12 patients treated with the stent-graft.

The endoluminal approach is cost-effective and the hospital and intensive care unit stay is much shorter. Acute type B dissections are the most appropriate group to treat, since the dissection flap will appose the aortic wall as the false lumen is excluded. Reperfusion of the branch vessels may then occur via the natural fenestrations in the flap corresponding to the original branch vessel ostia.

Combined technique for extensive dissection

A combination of surgery and percutaneous intervention may be employed in complex thoracic aortic pathology. The elephant trunk technique was first developed for the treatment of extensive thoracic aneurysm. In aortic dissection, experience with this particular stent-graft which doesn't necessarily require distal attachment has been reported. In one study, 22 patients (mean age 59 years) were treated: 12 type A dissection (3 acute, 9 chronic), 3 with type B dissection, and 7 with 'non-A/non-B' dissections with retrograde arch extension (or entry site in arch without ascending aortic involvement). All had aneurysms of the descending or thoraco-abdominal aorta. Patients underwent general anaesthesia under hypothermic circulatory arrest (15–20°C); 3 had anterograde cerebral perfusion, 6 had coronary bypass grafting or aortic valve replacement, 13 had a need for supra-aortic vessel bypass all without immediate complication. This technique allows complex aortic arch and descending thoracic dissection to be treated effectively with a significant reduction in operative risk. It remains likely that further technical developments will ultimately lead to percutaneous treatment for ascending aortic dissection as well.

Key points

- Acute aortic dissection in a high mortality condition with a 48-hour mortality of 50 per cent, with 70 per cent dead at 1 week and 90 per cent dead at 3 months, if left untreated. With treatment, overall hospital mortality is 27 per cent.
- Acute thoracic dissection is strongly associated with systemic hypertension and with advancing age. Several connective tissue disorders (of which Marfan's syndrome is the commonest) are

associated with dissection due to cystic medial degeneration in the aortic wall.

- There are pathological variations accounting for one-eighth of cases of 'aortic dissection'. In penetrating atherosclerotic ulcers (PAU), no intimal flap is demonstrable with a crater visible extending into the aortic wall associated with haematoma within the media of the aortic wall. Intramural haematoma (IMH) occurs where significant thickening or enhancement of the aortic wall is seen in the absence of a flap or dissection.

- Aortic dissection can mimic different conditions in the evolution of the symptoms and signs such as severe chest pain, vasovagal symptoms and hypotension, severe hypertension, acute aortic regurgitation, myocardial infarction, stroke, pleural effusion and visceral infarction.

- The diagnosis is most accurately done with spiral computed tomography (with contrast enhancement), although transoesophageal echography (TOE) is an alternative in many environments as it is portable, rapidly performed, sensitive and specific, and does not require the use of contrast agents. Magnetic resonance imaging (MRI) gives an improved anatomic delineation of the aorta and can provide high quality images in several planes.

- Patients in whom thoracic aortic dissection is suspected should be monitored and treated in a high dependency environment, and prepared for the possibility of early surgery. The two initial goals of therapy are pain relief and the reduction of the systolic pressure to a range of 100–120 mmHg (equivalent to a mean arterial pressure of 60–75 mmHg and sufficient to maintain vital organ perfusion). Where possible, left ventricular contractility should be reduced by beta-blockade independently of systemic blood pressure lowering.

- Urgent surgery is indicated in ascending thoracic aortic dissection and in descending thoracic aortic dissection where there are complications such as visceral ischaemia, threatened rupture, and retrograde dissection to ascending aorta.

- The use of percutaneous stent-graft technology to treat type B dissections is the major growth area in aortic dissection management.

Key references

Anangostopoulos CE, Prabhakar MJS, Kittle CF. Aortic dissections and dissecting aneurysms. *Am J Cardiol* 1972; **30**: 263–73.

Cambria RP, Brewster DC, Gertler J *et al.* Vascular complications associated with spontaneous aortic dissection. *J Vasc Surg* 1988; **7**: 199–209.

Casselaman FP, Tan ES, Vermeulen FE *et al.* Durability of aortic valve preservation and root reconstruction in acute type A aortic dissection. *Ann Thorac Surg* 2000; **70**: 1227–33.

Coady MA, Rizzo JA, Elefteriades JA. Pathologic variants of thoracic aortic dissections: penetrating atherosclerotic ulcers and intramural hematomas. *Cardiol Clin* 1999; **17**: 637–57.

Daily PO, Trueblood HW, Stinson EB, Wuerflein RD, Shumway NE. Management of acute aortic dissection. *Ann Thorac Surg* 1970; **10**: 237–47.

Dake MD, Kato N, Mitchell S *et al.* Endovascular stent-graft placement for the treatment of acute aortic dissection. *N Engl J Med* 1999; **340**: 1546–52.

DeBakey ME, McCollum CH, Crawford ES *et al.* Dissection and dissecting aneurysms of the aorta: 20-year follow-up of 527 patients treated surgically. *Surgery* 1982; **92**: 1118–34.

Doroghazi RM, Slater EE, DeSanctis RW *et al.* Long-term survival of patients with treated aortic dissection. *J Am Coll Cardiol* 1984; **3**: 1026–34.

Erbel R, Oelert H, Meyer J *et al.* Effect of medical and surgical therapy on aortic dissection evaluated by transoesophageal echocardiography. Implications for prognosis and therapy. *Circulation* 1993; **87**: 1604–15.

Ergin MA, Phillips RA, Galla JD *et al.* Significance of distal false lumen after type A dissection repair. *Ann Thorac Surg* 1994; **57**: 820–5.

Hagan PG, Nienaber CA, Isselbacher EM *et al.* The International Registry of Acute Aortic Dissection (IRAD). New insights into an old disease. *JAMA* 2000; **283**: 897–903.

Heinemann M, Laas J, Karck M, Borst HG. Thoracic aortic aneurysms after type A aortic dissection: necessity for follow-up. *Ann Thorac Surg* 1990; **49**: 580–4.

Kaji S, Nishigami K, Akasada T *et al.* Prediction of progression or regression of type A aortic intramural hematoma by computed tomography. *Circulation* 1999; **100**(Suppl 19): II281–6.

Khandheria BK. Aortic dissection. The last frontier. *Circulation* 1993; **87**: 1765–7.

Kieffer E, Koskas F, Godet G *et al.* Treatment of aortic arch dissection using the elephant trunk technique. *Ann Vasc Surg* 2000; **14**: 612–19.

Kolff J, Bates RJ, Balderman SC, Shenkoya K, Anagnostopoulos CE. Acute aortic arch dissection: re-evaluation of the indication for medical and surgical therapy. *Am J Cardiol* 1977; **39**: 727–33.

Masuda Y, Yamada Z, Morooka N, Watanabe S, Inagaki Y. Prognosis of patients with medically treated dissections. *Circulation* 1991; **84**: III7–13.

Miller DC. The continuing dilemma concerning medical versus surgical management of patients with acute type B dissections. *Semin Thorac Cardiovasc Surg* 1993; **5**: 33–46.

Miller DC, Stinson EB, Oyer PE *et al.* Operative treatment of aortic dissections. Experience with 125 patients over a sixteen-year period. *J Thorac Cardiovasc Surg* 1979; **78**: 365–81.

Moriyama Y, Yotsumoto G, Kuriwaki K *et al.* Intramural haematoma of the thoracic aorta. *Eur J Cardiothorac Surg* 1998; **13**: 230–9.

Nienaber CA, Fattori R, Lund G *et al*. Nonsurgical reconstruction of thoracic aortic dissection by stent-graft placement. *N Engl J Med* 1999; **340**: 1539–45.

Nienaber CA, von Kodolitsch Y, Petersen B *et al*. Intramural haemorrhage of the thoracic aorta: diagnostic and therapeutic implications. *Circulation* 1995; **92**: 1465–72.

Paneton JM, The SH, Cherry KJ *et al*. Aortic fenestration for acute or chronic aortic dissection. *J Vasc Surg* 2000; **32**: 711–21.

Pate JW, Richardson RJ, Eastridge CE. Acute aortic dissection. *Ann Surg* 1976; **42**: 395–404.

Rapezi C, Rocchi G, Fattori R *et al*. Usefulness of transoesophageal echocardiographic monitoring to improve the outcome of stent-graft treatment of thoracic aortic aneurysms. *Am J Cardiol* 2001; **87**: 315–19.

Slonim SM, Miller DC, Mitchell RS *et al*. Percutaneous balloon fenestration and stenting for life-threatening ischemic complications in patients with acute aortic dissection. *J Thorac Cardiovasc Surg* 1999; **117**: 1118–27.

Vilacosta I, San Roman JA, Ferreiros J *et al*. Natural history and serial morphology of aortic intramural haematoma: a novel variant of aortic dissection. *Am Heart J* 1997; **13**: 495–507.

Yamada T, Tada S, Harada J. Aortic dissection without intimal rupture: diagnosis with MR imaging and CT. *Radiology* 1988; **168**: 347–52.

Yucel EK, Steinberg FL, Egglin TK, Geller SC, Waltman AC, Athanasoulis CA. Penetrating aortic ulcers: diagnosis with MR imaging. *Radiology* 1990; **177**: 779–81.

Pulmonary embolism

Background

Epidemiology

Pulmonary embolism (PE) is a great constant in acute medicine with no major difference in its incidence or mortality in the past 20 years. It is unrecognized in the majority of cases and there is a direct relationship between age and mortality. Mortality is at least 10 per cent in the first few hours of presentation and the majority of patients with massive PE who die do not necessarily have specific symptoms to aid diagnosis.

Pathophysiology of venous thromboembolism

The mechanism of PE is through dislodgement of a venous thrombus from the deep veins of the leg or the pelvic veins into the pulmonary arterial circulation. The clinical signs produced by an embolism are determined by the level at which the thrombus is occlusive and to what extent pulmonary blood flow is diminished. Additional determinants of the clinical effect of embolism are the pre-existing cardiorespiratory reserve of the patient and the humoral effect of vasoactive factors such as serotonin and thromboxane A_2 released by activated platelets at the site of pulmonary artery occlusion. These peptides have a direct bronchoconstrictor effect in addition to a vasoconstrictor action. The risk of pulmonary embolism with a proximal deep venous thrombosis above the calf is as high as 50 per cent, with a lower risk in thromboses confined to the calf.

The development of a venous thrombus is initiated by Virchow's triad of local injury, hypercoagulability and stasis of flow. A hypercoagulable state is commonly acquired and thus secondary although there are a few rare primary conditions that predispose to a venous thrombus, usually in a younger age group ($<$45 years old) with an unexpected thromboembolism. Such hypercoagulable conditions exist in antithrombin III deficiency, protein C deficiency, protein S deficiency, and in inherited conditions with defective tPA (tissue plasminogen activator) release. The presence of the 'lupus anticoagulant' (with or without systemic lupus), which interferes with phospholipid-dependent coagulation, is associated with venous thrombosis. Some of these patients have anticardiolipin antibodies, which paradoxically prolong the activated partial thromboplastin time (aPTT). It is much commoner to see venous thromboembolism in clinical situations associated with abnormalities in coagulation, platelet function, or venous blood flow. The commonest clinical situations increasing risk for PE through promoting coagulation are:

- after surgery, particularly orthopaedic procedures;
- in cancer, with venous thrombosis often occurring before overt malignancy;
- altered hormonal state, such as the early post-partum period in pre-eclampsia as well as the rare association with the oral contraceptive pill.

Platelet aggregation may be enhanced in heparin-induced thrombocytopenia and in myeloproliferative disorders leading to thrombosis. Similarly, patients with hyperviscosity syndromes (polycythaemia, leukaemia and sickle cell disease) are more likely to have thrombotic complications. Venous thrombosis is common in the nephrotic syndrome.

Venous stasis may also be promoted by mechanical variables such as immobilization with chronic illness and obesity. Prolonged central venous cannulation for long-term drug therapy or parenteral nutrition can lead to right atrial thrombus formation and subsequent embolism. The relative risk of pulmonary embolism in different clinical situations is detailed in Table 7.1.

Table 7.1 Incidence of pulmonary embolism in different clinical situations

Clinical situation	Low risk	Intermediate risk	High risk
General surgery	Age <40 years Surgery <30 min No risk factors	Age 40–60 years Surgery 30–60 min	Age >60 years Surgery >60 min + risk factors
Orthopaedic surgery	Minor trauma	Leg plaster cast	Hip/knee surgery Hip fracture Multiple trauma
Medical conditions	Pregnancy	Heart failure Stroke Malignancy	Prolonged immobility
Incidence (Percentage)			
Distal DVT	2	10–40	40–80
Proximal DVT	0.4	6–8	10–15
Symptomatic PE	0.2	1–2	5–10
Fatal PE	0.002	0.1–0.8	1–5

Adapted from Riedel M. Acute pulmonary embolism. 2: Treatment. *Heart* 2001; **85**: 351–60.

Diagnosis of deep venous thrombosis

Diagnosis of deep venous thrombosis (DVT) is often difficult, and frequently missed. The clinical suspicion of a DVT (leg swelling, calf tenderness, venous distension of subcutaneous vessels, discoloration) should be confirmed objectively. This is necessary due to the lack of predictive accuracy in the clinical examination: calf pain has 66–91 per cent sensitivity and a 30–87 per cent specificity for DVT. A variety of investigations are available to confirm or rule out a diagnosis of DVT.

Contrast venography

Because of improvements in ultrasound resolution, the need for venography has diminished and it should be reserved for situations where the ultrasound examination is equivocal or normal where a high clinical suspicion still persists. With large extensive deep thromboses, the contrast injected in the foot may not reach the deep veins, leading to a false-negative venogram. The most reliable criterion for the diagnosis of acute DVT is a constant intraluminal filling defect evident in two or more views. An abrupt cut-off is reliable but may occur with previous DVT. Other criteria such as non-visualization of deep veins, venous collaterals, or non-constant intraluminal filling defects are less reliable. Disadvantages include its invasiveness, allergic reaction to dye and toxicity from the dye. The investigation itself may rarely cause a DVT through phlebitis. It is relatively contraindicated in acute renal failure and in critical peripheral vascular disease.

Impedance plethysmography (IPG)

This is a safe, non-invasive, operator-dependent, portable technique which evaluates the rate of venous return from the lower extremity. The test is based on the principle that the volume of blood in the leg affects its ability to conduct an applied current (inversely proportional to the impedance in two limb electrodes). A small current is passed between two electrodes with a second pair measuring voltage. Venous outflow is obstructed by a thigh cuff, which causes a fall-off in impedance. Once venous pressure reaches equilibrium, an increase in proximal blood flow occurs with the release of the cuff, increasing impedance. If a DVT is present in a major vein from the popliteals to the iliacs, the rate of venous emptying (and increase in impedance) is slower. This technique is insensitive to most calf thrombi and small non-obstructing proximal thrombi which do not decrease the rate of venous outflow, and false positives may also occur where a high central venous pressure is present, in massive obesity, reduced arterial perfusion, with non-thrombotic venous outflow obstruction such as in pregnancy and with pelvic masses.

Studies have demonstrated sensitivities of 92–98 per cent for symptomatic proximal DVT, compared to a sensitivity of only 20 per cent for calf DVT. Serial IPG studies over a 2-week period can demonstrate proximal extension in around 5 per cent of patients (test conversion from negative to positive). Negative IPG has been associated with a small rate of subsequent PE of around 2.5 per cent.

Compression ultrasound with venous imaging

The combination of colour doppler measurement of venous flow with two-dimensional cross-sectional assessment of lower extremity veins is termed duplex ultrasound. As with IPG, it is non-invasive and portable and has the ability to identify other causes of calf/thigh symptoms such as Baker's cysts, haematomas, lymphadenopathy, femoral artery aneurysm, superficial thrombophlebitis and abscesses. Pressure is applied with the ultrasound transducer to compress opposing venous walls with the primary diagnostic criterion being the non-compressibility of a vein. The presence of intraluminal echogenic thrombus, venous distension, absence of a colour flow doppler signal, and loss of phasic flow are secondary criteria. Its diagnostic accuracy is limited in pelvic and calf DVT and in asymptomatic proximal DVT, as well as in the presence of severe obesity or oedema. Acute DVT may be differentiated from chronic DVT by an increased compressibility and reduced echogenicity of thrombus seen. Ultrasound may not return to normal after a DVT and may be less useful for diagnosing recurrent DVT.

For proximal DVT, a sensitivity of 89–100 per cent and specificity of 95–100 per cent is reported with ultrasound. On balance, whether B-mode compression, duplex ultrasound or colour flow doppler is used, the positive and negative predictive accuracy is similar. Because calf veins are smaller and characterized by slower flow, and are more anatomically variable than the more proximal veins, ultrasound assessment is more difficult. Sensitivity ranges from 73 to 87 per cent with a specificity of 83–100 per cent, dropping to a sensitivity of 33–58 per cent in asymptomatic calf DVT.

Magnetic resonance imaging (MRI)

MRI has a high sensitivity for thrombus (up to 100 per cent) and allows assessment of the pelvic veins and inferior vena cava (IVC) in addition to the proximal veins in the thigh. Compared to contrast venography, it is less sensitive for calf DVT. It is non-invasive and not operator-dependent (but reader-dependent) and allows assessment of extraneous pathologies. It is more expensive than other technologies and is precluded by metallic objects and massive obesity/claustrophobia.

In summary, in the presence of a suspected acute DVT, either compression ultrasound or IPG should be done. If inconclusive or inadequate, venography or MRI should be done. If the initial assessment is normal and the patient can return for a repeat study, serial ultrasound or IPG may be done over a period of 7–14 days. If the patient cannot return, if iliac vein thrombosis is suspected, or if an urgent diagnosis is deemed necessary, venography (or MRI) should be done.

Clinical presentation

Acute minor PE

It is estimated that about 40 per cent of patients with a deep venous thrombosis who have no pulmonary symptoms have abnormal lung scintigrams indicating embolism. Thus, many minor PEs remain asymptomatic. In the 10 per cent of these patients who obstruct a branch pulmonary artery, pulmonary infarction will occur with sudden dyspnoea and usually sharp pleuritic pain associated with haemoptysis. The incidence of infarction is higher in the presence of chronic respiratory or cardiac disease. In minor embolism, there will be no central cyanosis due to relatively insignificant ventilation/perfusion mismatch and normal right ventricular function with preservation of the cardiac output.

Acute massive PE

A large clot occluding a major pulmonary artery or partially obstructing the main pulmonary artery (>50 per cent of the pulmonary vascular bed) will result in an acute increase in right ventricular afterload and an elevation in pulmonary artery pressure with an increased likelihood of a sudden cardiac death. The commonest clinical features in this situation are syncope (often in the context of paradoxical bradycardia), acute severe dyspnoea, acute right heart failure, cardiogenic shock and cardiac arrest with electromechanical dissociation. Significant cardiorespiratory compromise leads to a sinus tachycardia, tachypnoea and central cyanosis through ventilation/perfusion mismatch. To maintain cardiac output, the pulmonary artery pressure rises with consequent pressure load (up to 55 mmHg) on the right ventricle, increasing right ventricular work.

In otherwise fit patients, once more than 25 per cent of the pulmonary vascular bed is occluded, there is an increased afterload or pressure load on the right ventricle, leading to an increase in right ventricular systolic pressure. With increasing pressure load, the right ventricle will dilate (against a restrictive pericardium) with the development of functional tricuspid regurgitation, an increased right atrial pressure and, ultimately, cardiogenic shock. The paradoxical movement of a pressure-loaded right ventricle leads to left ventricular diastolic dysfunction in addition to a reduction in left ventricular preload through a reduced transpulmonary blood flow. Echocardiography identifies these features with an increase in right ventricular end-systolic and end-diastolic diameters and septal flattening in both phases of the cardiac cycle. Left ventricular end-diastolic diameter is also reduced with significant embolism.

The mechanism of hypoxaemia in massive PE is multifactorial. It occurs through significant ventilation/perfusion mismatch, and may also occur due to intrapulmonary arteriovenous (AV) shunting through areas poorly ventilated with residual blood flow. Shunting may also occur at an atrial level where acute right heart pressures may reverse flow through a patent foramen ovale. Where the cardiac output is low, insufficient gas exchange may occur in the residual areas of perfusion, leading to further systemic desaturation. Hypercapnia is rare in massive PE due to tachypnoea.

Symptoms of massive PE are severe dyspnoea (not orthopnoea), syncope and low cardiac output. Angina may occur through a combination of hypoxaemia, tachycardia and hypotension. Central cyanosis and acute right heart strain ensue. It may be difficult to hear a right ventricular gallop rhythm or widely split second heart sound in the presence of significant respiratory distress.

Diagnosis of acute pulmonary embolism

The need for objective testing is necessary as the diagnosis of PE is difficult on clinical grounds. Unexplained dyspnoea, pleuritic chest pain and haemoptysis are classical symptoms with tachypnoea in particular and tachycardia being common signs but all are non-specific. Similarly, syncope or sudden hypotension may indicate a large clot burden but can be due to different causes. The differential diagnosis of acute PE includes:

- acute coronary syndrome (particularly MI)
- acute proximal aortic dissection
- acute pulmonary oedema
- acute pneumonia
- pleurisy
- acute bronchospasm
- acute exacerbations of chronic airflow limitation
- bronchogenic carcinoma
- pneumothorax
- chest wall syndrome
- fractured rib.

Because of the difficulty in establishing a diagnosis of PE on clinical grounds, it is vital to employ a combination of simple [electrocardiogram (ECG), chest x-ray, echocardiography, blood gases, D-dimer] and complex [ventilation/perfusion (V/Q) scan, computed tomography (CT), MRI, angiography] investigations to confirm a clinical suspicion.

12-lead ECG

Although 87 per cent of patients have an abnormal ECG, these largely include T-wave changes, ST segment abnormalities, and left or right axis deviation. In the Urokinase Pulmonary Embolism Trial (UPET), 32 per cent if patients with massive PE and 26 per cent of those with massive/submassive PE had ECG signs of acute cor pulmonale such as the $S_1Q_3T_3$ pattern, right bundle branch block, P pulmonale or right axis deviation.

Arterial blood gases

Hypoxaemia is very common but not universally present. In one study, a Po_2 of >11 kPa was found in 29 per cent of patients younger than 40 compared to only 3 per cent of older patients. Hypoxia is more common in patients with pre-existing cardiorespiratory disease.

Chest radiography

Common non-specific radiographic appearances are atelectasis, pleural effusion, infiltrates and an effusion. Decreased vacscularity is uncommon. The presence of a normal chest x-ray in the presence of hypoxaemia in the absence of an intracardiac shunt or bronchospasm is highly suggestive of PE. The value of a chest x-ray is that it allows exclusion of other pathological processes such as pneumonia, pneumothorax or rib fracture.

D-dimer

When cross-linked fibrin undergoes fibrinolysis, D-dimers are released and can be measured by an enzyme-linked immunoadsorbent assay (ELISA) or latex agglutination test. A low plasma D-dimer concentration (<500 μg/L) has a 95 per cent negative predictive accuracy. In one study of 308 patients presenting acutely with suspected PE, patients underwent assessment of clinical probability, ventilation/perfusion scan, D-dimer, and lower extremity ultrasound. Of 198 patients with suspected embolism and a D-dimer level <500 μg/L, 196 were free of PE, with one actual event (and one lost to follow-up). The accuracy of rapid bedside D-dimer testing is still under investigation.

Ventilation/perfusion scan

Although a common test of pulmonary embolism, the V/Q scan is quite non-specific and is diagnostic (normal or high probability) in a minority

Table 7.2 Clinical assessment and ventilation/perfusion scan probability

	Clinical probability (in percentage)		
V/Q scan (probability)	Highly likely (80–100)	Uncertain (20–79)	Unlikely (0–19)
High	96	88	56
Intermediate	66	28	16
Low	40	16	4
Near normal/normal	0	6	2
Total	68	30	9

of cases. In the PIOPED study, which validated the V/Q scan against pulmonary angiography or post-mortem, it was apparent that PE was present in the presence of non-diagnostic scans in 40 per cent of cases (Table 7.2).

With increasing background cardiorespiratory disease, the V/Q scan becomes less helpful with an increase in intermediate-probability scans, particularly with the coexistence of chronic obstructive airways disease (60 per cent of scans are intermediate-probability). If a ventilation scan cannot be performed, an isolated perfusion scan is useful if it is high probability, low probability, near normal or normal. In the interpretation of perfusion scans, it is imperative that one or more segmental perfusion defects are considered diagnostic of embolism. When the lung scan is non-diagnostic, evaluation of the lower extremities is an alternative means by which to assess the need for anticoagulation. In general, treatment for patients should be individualized. With a near-normal or low-probability scan, and a negative leg study (by ultrasound or plethysmography), and a low clinical suspicion, no treatment is needed. With a low-probability scan and negative leg study, but an uncertain or high clinical suspicion, the PE estimate is between 9 and 25 per cent. With intermediate-probability scans, but a negative leg study, either pulmonary angiography or serial non-invasive leg studies should be done, depending on the stability of the patient. In one study to evaluate the latter course, stability was defined as absence of pulmonary oedema, right ventricular failure, systolic blood pressure < 90 mmHg, syncope, tachydysrhythmia, $FEV_1 < 1.0$ l, FVC < 1.5 L, $Po_2 < 7$ kPa, and $Pco_2 > 6$ kPa. Of 627 patients with non-diagnostic lung scans and negative serial plethysmography in whom treatment was withheld, only 1.9 per cent had a venous thromboembolic complication. This compares with 0.7 per cent of untreated patients with normal lung scans and 5.5 per cent of high-probability scans who received treatment.

Pulmonary angiography

Pulmonary angiography is the invasive gold standard for diagnosing PE and has been used where a ventilation scan is non-diagnostic. It involves passing a pigtail catheter percutaneously to the main pulmonary artery with selective and sub-selective dye injections into the pulmonary circulation under fluoroscopic imaging. A positive finding is an intraluminal filling defect in two views and the demonstration of an occluded pulmonary artery with or without a trailing edge. Less specific criteria are reduced perfusion, abnormal parenchymal stain and a delayed venous return. In the PIOPED study, where 1111 pulmonary angiograms were performed, 35 per cent were positive, 61 per cent were negative, with 3 per cent non-diagnostic and 1 per cent non-completion. In small PE, the reliability of angiography is reduced. The mortality of pulmonary angiography is 0.5 per cent with severe cardiopulmonary compromise in 0.4 per cent, and morbidity tends to be higher in critically ill patients from intensive care. This technique requires invasive expertise but may be an appropriate investigation in patients with massive PE who are candidates for percutaneous intervention to the pulmonary thrombus.

Spiral computed tomography

This technique allows rapid tomographic imaging with continuous volume acquisition during a single breath-hold. The pulmonary vasculature may be visualized with a contrast dye injection (CT pulmonary angiogram). The technique is limited by poorer visualization of the peripheral areas of the upper and lower lobes. In comparative studies, spiral CT is associated with 95 per cent specificity and sensitivity for PE. Spiral CT has the greatest sensitivity for emboli in the main, lobar or segmental pulmonary arteries with a reduced sensitivity in the subsegmental branches, e.g. a pick-up rate of 25–30 per cent. There is some evidence that thinner slice CT images and two-dimensional reformation of the scan may enhance sensitivity. An additional advantage of spiral CT is the ability to define non-vascular structures such as lymphadenopathy, lung tumours and emphysema and other parenchymal and pleural disease. The high specificity of spiral CT is reader-dependent. The general feeling in practice is that it is best deployed as a confirmatory technique rather than a screening test. Breath-holding is unnecessary with electron beam (ultrafast) CT with a minimizing of cardiac and respiratory movement. In comparison with pulmonary angiography, only 1 per cent of vascular zones are inadequately visualized.

MRI

With experienced readers, the sensitivity and specificity of MRI to detect PE is 73 per cent and 97 per cent, respectively (with the potential to improve sensitivity with gadolinium injection). The technique is more rapid, less invasive and avoids nephrotoxic contrast compared to pulmonary angiography. There is a lesser evidence base for MRI than for CT at present but given its proven ability to detect leg vein thrombi (along with lung perfusion imaging), there is an obvious appeal for a combined technique.

Echocardiography

Right ventricular failure frequently accompanies massive PE and correlates with larger emboli and with the recurrence of PE. Other causes of pulmonary hypertension may also produce this appearance, however. Akinesis of the mid-free wall with apical sparing may be more common in acute PE (77 per cent sensitivity, 94 per cent specificity). Conversely, massive PE may be associated with good right ventricular function. Transoesophageal echocardiography may permit visualization of massive emboli in the proximal pulmonary arteries, which may be enhanced by contrast. The quality of the imaging will be limited by chronic airflow limitation and obesity.

An important role of echocardiography is its use to exclude alternative cases of acute cardiorespiratory compromise such as aortic dissection, acute ventricular septal rupture, large MI or cardiac tamponade.

Acute treatment of pulmonary embolism

The overriding strategy in the treatment of PE is the reduction of thrombosis, both the development and propagation of venous thrombus and the fibrinolysis or break-up of established, embolized clot. With the acute presentation of a PE, it is imperative that the diagnosis is made quickly and an assessment of the patient's haemodynamic state made. The primary therapies are:

- heparin 5000–10 000 units. This may be initiated at the start of the diagnostic process.
- oxygen supplementation, initially by face mask although supportive ventilation may be necessary.

- haemodynamic support. Noradrenaline may be used in small doses to support the acute failure of the right ventricle, but only where the patient is in cardiogenic shock as it may be counterproductive with respect to cardiac rhythm. Right heart filling pressure should be supported to maintain right ventricular stroke volume, although this is finely balanced as volume loading may exacerbate paradoxical septal motion, leading to a reduction in left ventricular stroke volume.

In the absence of circulatory failure, a strategy of anticoagulation is required. With haemodynamic compromise, thrombolysis and/or clot fragmentation is required.

Unfractionated heparin

The heparin–antithrombin III complex inactivates thrombin and to a lesser extent, activated factors IX and X. The efficacy of heparin in PE is through prevention of further fibrin generation from thrombin activation, this allowing the endogenous fibrinolytic system to dissolve residual thrombus. Unfractionated heparin (UFH) should be given early to achieve an adequate plasma concentration and through this and subsequent oral anticoagulation, the risk of recurrent venous thromboembolism and death is considerably reduced. By convention, UFH is given by initial bolus and intravenous infusion or subcutaneously (given as 250 U/kg b.d. to achieve adequate anticoagulation. If the activated partial thromboplastin time (aPTT) is prolonged prior to heparin therapy, antiphospholipid antibodies should be considered as a pro-thrombotic influence (and direct anticoagulation managed by the heparin level itself rather than by aPTT monitoring). Rarely, antithrombin III deficiency will lead to true heparin resistance.

The problem with UFH is its unpredictable haematological response due to the binding of heparin to plasma and endothelial proteins, regardless of weight adjustment. To control for this, the aPTT should also be measured 4–6 hours after initiation and similarly after any dose change to be maintained at 1.5–2.5 mean control value. Oral anticoagulation should be started simultaneously with heparin discontinued once the international normalized ratio (INR) is >2.0 on two consecutive days. Serious complications from heparin therapy occur in less than 5 per cent of patients and are more common where there is an existing bleeding diathesis or pathology such as active or previous peptic ulcer disease/varices/angiodysplasia, recent surgery, severe hypertension, or recent haemorrhagic stroke. Long-term (>2 months) heparin therapy is associated with osteoporosis and skin rashes and hypersensitivity reactions can occur. Mild heparin-induced thrombocytopenia (HIT) may occur within the first few days of treatment due to direct aggregation. When it occurs after the first 5–7 days, due to antibody formation it is more severe (platelet count $< 100 \times 10^9/\text{L}$). Heparin should be discontinued with substitution by a direct antithrombin drug, e.g. hirudin, as significant pro-thrombotic risk exists. This HIT with thrombosis is very serious and any potential effect of heparin on platelets should be monitored with immediate discontinuation if the platelet count drops.

Low molecular weight heparin (LMWH)

LMWH has become the treatment of choice for venous thromboembolism. It is produced by depolymerization of unfractionated heparin, leading to small molecules capable of inhibiting activated factor X in preference to thrombin (activated factor II). Given a longer half-life and less ancillary binding, the anticoagulant dose is predictable after subcutaneous dosing. As the aPTT measures antithrombin activity, LMWH anticoagulation should, if necessary, be monitored by its anti-Xa activity. Its administration subcutaneously requires less supervision and may be given once or twice daily (depending on exact LMWH type) to give as effective a therapy as UFH in the treatment of proximal DVT and acute PE. Its role in massive PE is less well validated, however.

Thrombolytic therapy

Thrombolytic therapy is indicated in the treatment of massive PE (shock, severe hypoxaemia) or PE with echocardiographic evidence of right ventricular dysfunction. Thrombolytic therapy actively promotes fibrinolysis. Because of this, it has additional benefit in breaking up residual deep venous thrombus and reduces the risk of recurrent PE and chronic thromboembolism. Several thrombolytic agents have been used (streptokinase, urokinase, and the more fibrin-specific tissue plasminogen activators and reteplase), which work through different means to convert plasminogen to plasmin, which degrades fibrin in clot. All appear to be equally effective and safe. However, despite the appeal, no large randomized trials of thrombolytic therapy against heparin powered to demonstrate a difference in hard clinical outcomes exist. This is because of the relatively low mortality of PE and the fact that patients with large emboli entering a trial have self-selected themselves as a good prognostic group. Improvements in clinical stability and perfusion scans with early resolution of emboli have been reported with thrombolysis. In one non-randomized comparison of thrombolysis ($n = 169$) with UFH

($n = 550$) in non-shocked patients, 30-day mortality was lower with thrombolysis, 4.7 per cent vs 11.1 per cent, as was recurrent PE, 7.7 per cent vs 18.7 per cent.

Contraindications to thrombolytic therapy are similar to those in the treatment of MI, but by contrast, intravenous thrombolysis is effective for up to 2 weeks after presentation. The risk of bleeding is greatest where the administration of thrombolysis is prolonged or where vascular puncture sites are present. If persistent major bleeding occurs, plasmin activity can be reversed by intravenous aprotinin and fibrinogen replenished with clotting factors in fresh frozen plasma (which will contain plasminogen).

Suggested doses for thrombolytic drugs for pulmonary embolism are:

- streptokinase 0.25–0.5 MU over 15 minutes followed by 0.1 MU/h for 24 hours;
- urokinase 4400 U/kg over 10 minutes then 4400 U/kg for 12 hours;
- tPA 10 mg bolus, then 90 mg over 2 hours;
- reteplase two 10 U boluses 30 minutes apart.

Recent studies show no excess of fatal bleeding compared with conventional treatment with heparin.

Surgical pulmonary embolectomy

The rapid restoration of pulmonary blood flow is likely to be a major determinant in preventing mortality from massive PE. In the past, surgery was considered the best means of removing significant clot load. The vogue for surgical embolectomy even in extreme situations is diminishing. Historically, patients in shock despite inotropic support who continue to deteriorate and those with major contraindications to thrombolysis have been considered for surgical embolectomy. Retrospective series largely predate the use of thrombolysis and include procedures outside the emergency setting. High operative mortality of up to 50 per cent has been reported, and current practice has included femoral-to-femoral bypass for haemodynamic support prior to full cardiopulmonary bypass. The need for cardiopulmonary resuscitation prior to surgery predicts an adverse outcome from surgical embolectomy. With survival from the procedure, most late morbidity is neurological.

Mechanical thrombectomy

In the modern era of percutaneous intervention, attempts have been made to provide an alternative to surgical embolectomy. Initial techniques have focused on retrieval devices to hold and extract a thrombus from the main pulmonary artery in patients with massive pulmonary embolism. However, this approach has had limited success. Clot fragmentation has been described in uncontrolled studies using a pigtail or Judkins catheter. The theoretical benefit of this approach is that the clot will fragment into a smaller vascular area as it embolizes distally and will be more susceptible to thrombolysis. This will reduce pulmonary artery pressure and improve transpulmonary flow in most cases. In cases where PA pressure remains high, this may occur through release of vasoconstrictor hormones such as thromboxane A_2, arguing for the actual removal of clot rather than simple embolization of it. Again, outcome data for this technique are limited. However, newer devices are becoming available which both fragment and aspirate clot such as the Hydrolyser™, Amplatz™ and Günther catheters. The most promising device may be the Arrow–Trerotola percutaneous thrombolytic device (PTD) which consists of a motor-driven 5F outer catheter connected to a fragmentation basket which rotates at 3000 r.p.m. The latest version of this device may be introduced over the wire through a guide catheter into the thrombus and activated to fragment thrombus. Clinical studies are also ongoing with respect to the fragmentation of ileofemoral thrombus via the transjugular route using this device. It can be deployed in the pelvic veins with the adjunctive use of a temporarily deployed wall stent in the IVC to act as a filter for old thrombus which can then be removed back into a large 15F guide catheter.

Chronic treatment of pulmonary embolism

Oral anticoagulation for PE

It is imperative that warfarin is started soon after diagnosis is made and acute treatment started so that an overlap can occur for a period of 5 days to avoid the pro-thrombotic state created by a reduction in protein C with oral anticoagulation. The prothrombin time expressed as the INR should be adjusted to a therapeutic window of 2.0–3.0, or higher where the antiphospholipid syndrome is the cause of the embolism. In the medium-term treatment of the patient, obvious risk factors should be corrected which may allow a shorter period of anticoagulation compared to the standard period of 3–6 months for a first PE. In the presence of a persistent procoagulant stimulus such as malignant disease or proven thrombophilia or where recurrent PE has occurred (prior PE is the best predictor of recurrent DVT) or the patient had chronic thromboembolic disease, treatment should be prolonged or lifelong. Significant bleeding complications with over-anticoagulation should be treated with a bolus of 0.5–1.0 mg vitamin K which will bring the INR back into the normal range. This can take up to 24 hours so clotting factor concentrates or fresh frozen plasma should be given for quicker restoration of haemostasis.

Oral anticoagulation for DVT

Anticoagulation is required to reduce the risk of proximal propagation and embolism to the pulmonary circulation. DVT proximal to the calf and symptomatic calf (popliteal) DVTs require LMWH injections and an arbitrary 3-month course of warfarin. A 20 per cent recurrence rate has been reported in the literature. Patients with symptomatic DVT do not all require hospital admission and patients may be risk-stratified according to PE risk (see Table 7.1). Long-term anticoagulation is required in significantly obese patients and in those with cancer, and previous DVT. Anticoagulation is not mandatory in asymptomatic calf DVTs as long as serial ultrasound monitoring confirms no proximal extension. A majority of patients develop chronic venous insufficiency after anticoagulant therapy and the use of high pressure support stockings prevents venous wall distension on ambulation, which may reduce this risk.

Inferior vena caval filters

These filters can be introduced percutaneously to prevent significant thrombus reaching the pulmonary circulation. Their use should be restricted to situations where recurrent DVTs occur despite adequate anticoagulation or used in patients who cannot tolerate warfarin on a temporary or permanent basis. The long-term use of these devices has been associated with caval thrombosis at the filter site, filter fracture and migration and occasional vessel wall perforation.

Thromboembolic pulmonary disease

Patients with recurrent pulmonary emboli may go on to develop chronic thromboembolic disease with pulmonary hypertension and ultimately cor pulmonale. This occurs where recurrent PE has been undiagnosed over several weeks to months without oral antiocagulation. The best treatment option for this rare condition is surgical thromboendarterectomy with removal of organized clot ideally as a cast of the pulmonary vascular tree. As with acute surgical embolectomy, this operation carries a significant mortality and it is likely that a percutaneous thrombectomy technique will supersede this approach.

Key points

- Pulmonary embolism occurs through dislodgement of a venous thrombus from the deep leg or the pelvic veins into the pulmonary arterial circulation. The clinical signs of embolism are determined by the level at which the thrombus is occlusive.
- The development of a venous thrombus is determined by Virchow's triad of local injury, hypercoagulability and stasis of flow.
- Venous thromboembolism is a clinical situation where the diagnosis is more often not made than made. The clinical suspicion of a deep venous thrombosis (leg swelling, calf tenderness, venous distension of subcutaneous vessels, discoloration) should be confirmed objectively, due to the lack of predictive accuracy in the clinical examination.
- In the presence of a suspected acute deep venous thrombosis, either compression ultrasound or IPG should be done. If inconclusive or inadequate, venography or MRI should be done.
- In acute PE, classic symptoms are unexplained dyspnoea, pleuritic chest pain and haemoptysis with tachypnoea in particular and tachycardia being common signs but all are non-specific.
- The ventilation/perfusion (V/Q) scan is often non-specific and in one study which evaluated the V/Q scan by pulmonary angiography or post-mortem, it was apparent that PE was present in 40 per cent of patients with non-diagnostic scans.
- Pulmonary angiography is the invasive gold standard for diagnosing PE and may be used where a ventilation scan has been non-diagnostic. A positive finding is an intraluminal filling defect in two views and the demonstration of an occluded pulmonary artery.
- Computed tomography is limited by poorer visualization of the peripheral areas of the lung but is associated with 95 per cent specificity and sensitivity for PE. Spiral CT has the greatest sensitivity for emboli in the main, lobar or segmental pulmonary arteries.

- The acute treatment of PE includes intravenous heparin oxygen supplementation, and haemodynamic support with noradrenaline and careful volume balance. In the absence of circulatory failure, a strategy of anticoagulation is required. With haemodynamic compromise, thrombolysis and/or clot fragmentation is required.
- Clinical studies are ongoing with the percutaneous use of a thrombolytic device which consists of a motor-driven catheter connected to a fragmentation basket rotating at high speed. Other percutaneous devices use the Venturi effect to aspirate fresh clot both in the deep venous system and in the pulmonary circulation.

Key references

American Thoracic Society Statement. The diagnostic approach to acute venous thromboembolism. *Am J Respir Crit Care Med* 1999; **160**: 1043–66.

Bell WR, Simon TL, DeMets DL. The clinical features of submassive and massive pulmonary emboli. *Am J Med* 1977; **52**: 355–60.

Brady AJB, Crake T, Oakley CM. Percutaneous catheter fragmentation and distal dispersion of proximal pulmonary embolus. *Lancet* 1991; **338**: 1186–9.

Fava M, Loyola S, Flores P, Huete I. Mechanicla fragmentation and pharmacologic thrombolysis in massive pulmonary embolism. *J Vasc Intervent Radiol* 1997; **8**: 261–6.

Goldhaber SZ, Hennekens CH, Evans DA, Newton EC, Godleski JJ. Factors associated with correct antemortem diagnosis of major pulmonary embolism. *Am J Med* 1982; **73**: 822–6.

Goldhaber SZ, Markis JE, Meyerovitz MF *et al.* Acute pulmonary embolism treated with tissue plasminogen activator. *Lancet* 1986; **18**: 886–9.

Green RM, Meyer TJ, Dunn M, Glassroth J. Pulmonary embolism in younger adults. *Chest* 1992; **101**: 1507–11.

Greenfield LJ, Proctor MC, Williams DM, Wakefield TW. Long-term experience with transvenous catheter pulmonary embolectomy. *J Vasc Surg* 1993; **18**: 450–8.

Harrigan RA, Jones K. ABC of clinical electrocardiography. Conditions affecting the right side of the heart. *BMJ* 2002; **324**: 1201–4.

Hirsh J, Dalen JE, Anderson DR *et al.* Oral anticoagulants: mechanism of action, clinical effectiveness, and optimal therapeutic range. *Chest* 1998; **114**: 445S–69S.

Hull RD, Raskob G, Ginsberg JS *et al.* A noninvasive strategy for the treatment of patients with suspected pulmonary embolism. *Arch Intern Med* 1994; **154**: 289–97.

Konstantinides S, Geibel A, Olschewski M *et al.* Association between thrombolytic treatment and the prognosis of hemodynamically stable patients with major pulmonary embolism. Results of a multicenter registry. *Circulation* 1997; **96**: 882–8.

Konstantinides S, Giebel A, Heusel G *et al*. Heparin plus alteplase compared with heparin alone in patients with submassive pulmonary embolism. *N Engl J Med* 2002; **347**: 143–50.

Leclerc JR, Illescas F, Jarzem P. Diagnosis of deep vein thrombosis. In: Leclerc JR (ed.), *Venous Thromboembolic Disorders*. Philadelphia: Lea & Febiger, 1991: 176–228.

Moser KM, Daily PO, Peterson K *et al*. Thromboendarterectomy for chronic major-vessel thromboembolic pulmonary hypertension; immediate and long-term results in 42 patients. *Ann Intern Med* 1987; **107**: 560–5.

Perrier A, Bounameaux H, Morabia A *et al*. Diagnosis of pulmonary embolism by a decision analysis-based strategy including clinical probability, D-dimer levels, and ultrasonography: a management study. *Arch Intern Med* 1996; **156**: 531–6.

PIOPED investigators. Value of the ventilation-perfusion scan in acute pulmonary embolism: results of the Prospective Investigation of Pulmonary Embolism Diagnosis (PIOPED). *JAMA* 1990; **263**: 2753–9.

Raschke RA, Reilly BM, Guidry JR, Fontana JR, Srinivas S. The weight-based heparin dosing nomogram compared with a "standard care" nomogram. A randomized controlled trial. *Ann Intern Med* 1993; **119**: 874–81.

Ricek M, Peregrin J, Velimsky T. Mechanical thrombectomy of massive pulmonary embolism using an Arrow-Trerotola percutaneous thrombolytic device. *Eur Radiol* 1998; **8**; 163–5.

Riedel M. Acute pulmonary embolism. 1: Diagnosis. *Heart* 2001; **85**: 229–40.

Riedel M. Acute pulmonary embolism. 2: Treatment. *Heart* 2001; **85**: 351–60.

Riedel M. Therapy of pulmonary thromboembolism. Part 1: acute massive pulmonary embolism. *Cor Vasa* 1996; **38**: 93–102.

Urokinase Pulmonary Embolism Trial: a national co-operative study. *Circulation* 1973; **47**(Suppl II): 1–108.

Verstraete M, Miller GAH, Bounameaux H *et al*. Intravenous and intrapulmonary recombinant tissue-type plasminogen activator in the treatment of acute massive pulmonary embolism. *Circulation* 1988; **77**: 353–60.

Infective endocarditis

Background

Epidemiology and pathophysiology

Strictly speaking infective endocarditis (IE) is a disease in which an infective organism colonizes the heart valves, septal defects or mural endocardium. However, in clinical practice the definition extends to include infections on arteriovenous shunts, arterio-arterial shunts and aortic coarctations, as the clinical presentation is often indistinguishable. The infection evolves to produce a vegetation that comprises an amorphous mass of organisms, inflammatory cells, fibrin and platelets. Overall there are approximately 1500 cases of endocarditis in the UK per year, with an estimated in-patient mortality between 15 and 20 per cent. IE can occur not only on congenital or acquired structural cardiac abnormalities but also on normal, previously healthy valves. Traditionally, endocarditis has been divided into acute and subacute forms. Acute bacterial endocarditis is usually due to a virulent organism such as *Staphylococcus aureus*, which can rapidly lead to complications within days or weeks if left untreated.

Subacute bacterial endocarditis is more indolent, usually presents weeks to months after the initial infection and is caused by organisms such as *Streptococcus viridans* or coagulase-negative staphylococci. This classification was initially based on untreated disease. Since devastating complications such as valve perforation and cerebral embolization can arise with a variety of different organisms and bacteria are not always implicated, the term IE is more appropriate and is now widely used.

In the past, IE occurred mainly in patients with underlying rheumatic or congenital heart disease. As the incidence and prevalence of rheumatic heart disease has decreased in developed countries, IE affecting the native valves occurs largely in the setting of mitral valve prolapse, bicuspid or sclerotic aortic valves, degenerative mitral valve disease, congenital heart disease and intravenous drug abusers. Men are more likely to be affected than women and there is an increased incidence in the elderly population. Congenital heart disease is more important as a cause of IE in young adults. Mitral valve prolapse has emerged as an important structural cardiac lesion, accounting for up to one-third of cases of native valve endocarditis in adults, whereas degenerative heart disease is the main cause in the elderly (over the age of 60). Over the past years, intravenous drug abuse has become an important risk factor for the development of IE. It is usually associated with right-sided valve lesions, and can affect up to 7 per cent of intravenous drug abusers. *Staphylococcus aureus* is responsible for more than 50 per cent of these infections. Unusual organisms such as *Corynebacterium* species, *Bacillus cereus*, *Lactobacillus*, *Candida* and polymicrobial infections can sometimes be found in this population. In developed countries, epidemiological studies suggest that 10–20 per cent of patients with prosthetic heart valves develop endocarditis. The risk is greatest during the first 6 months after valve surgery and thereafter declines to about 0.2–0.35 per cent per year. The term 'early' is often used to describe prosthetic valve endocarditis when it occurs within 2 months following surgery, and is considered to be a complication of valve surgery. Prosthetic valve endocarditis occurring more than 12 months after surgery is termed 'late' and, like native valve endocarditis, is likely to be associated with community-acquired infections. Cases occurring between 2 and 12 months after surgery are a mixture of hospital-acquired episodes caused by less virulent organisms and community-acquired episodes. Hence, the timing of infection reflects different pathogenic mechanisms, which in turn influence the epidemiology, microbiology, pathology and clinical manifestation. The risk of invasive infection is increased among patients with prosthetic valve endocarditis within the first year after implantation, particularly those with infection of an aortic valve prosthesis. Table 8.1 summarizes the microbiology of IE in native and prosthetic heart valves, and in intravenous drug abusers.

Table 8.1 Microbiology of infective endocarditis

Organism	Non-addicts (%)	Addicts (%)	Early PVE (%)	Late PVE (%)
Streptococcus viridans	50	10	8	30
Enterococci	5	8	2	6
Other streptococci	5	2		
Staphylococcus aureus	20	57	15	10
Staphylococcus epidermidis	5	3	33	29
Gram-negative bacteria (including HACEK group)[a]	6	7	17	10
Fungus	1	5	10	5
Culture negative	5	5	5	5
Diphtheroids			8	3
Mixed/Others	3	3	2	2

[a] The HACEK group of organisms consists of *Haemophilus* species, *Actinobacillus* species, *Cardiobacterium* species, *Eikenella* species and *Kingella* species. These Gram-negative coccobacilli are fastidious and slow growing, and have become an important cause of IE. They are part of the respiratory tract and oropharyngeal flora.

The pathogenesis of IE involves turbulent blood flow from a high to a low pressure zone, resulting in damage to the endocardium and the formation of a sterile, platelet-fibrin thrombus. The presence of micro-organisms in the blood may then seed this thrombus and proliferate, resulting in IE. Vegetations are usually located along the line of closure of a valve leaflet on the low pressure side of the valve where turbulence occurs, that is, the atrial surface for atrioventricular valves or the ventricular surface for semilunar valves. The absence of a pressure gradient across an ostium secundum atrial septal defect explains the low risk of endocarditis in this group. Following successful treatment for IE, healing occurs by fibrosis and calcification.

Clinical presentation

The clinical syndrome of IE consists of fever, changing murmurs, septic embolization to any organ, and petechial lesions of the skin. The diagnosis should be suspected in anyone who presents with pyrexia and multi-system involvement, in the presence of cardiac disease or intravenous drug abuse.

Presentations may be acute, with a toxic, unwell patient with high fevers and rigors; subacute or chronic, which can present weeks or months after the initial infection, and can be associated with a low grade fever, night sweats, weight loss and anaemia (normochromic normocytic). Other associated symptoms and signs may include lethargy, anorexia, vague abdominal or flank pain, confusion, arthralgia, myalgia and finger clubbing. Peripheral manifestations as a result of an immunologically mediated vasculitis or septic embolization can give rise to:

- Osler's nodes (tender, subcutaneous nodules seen in the pulps of the digits);
- Janeway lesions (non-tender, erythematous or haemorrhagic macular lesions seen on the palms and soles);
- splinter haemorrhages in the fingernails or toenails; petechiae on the conjunctivae and buccal mucosa;
- focal glomerulonephritis and splenic infarcts;
- mycotic aneurysms and occlusion involving any vessel, commonly seen in the cerebral arteries, abdominal aorta, coronary arteries, gastrointestinal arteries, limb arteries and renal arterioles;
- retinal infarcts (Roth's spots), causing an oval-shaped haemorrhage with a pale centre;
- neurological involvement can occur in 30–40 per cent of patients with IE, the majority of which are embolic strokes, with intracranial haemorrhages occurring in 5 per cent;
- congestive cardiac failure as a result of valve destruction or rupture of a chorda and, rarely, intracardiac fistulae, myocarditis or coronary artery embolism;
- perivalvular extension beyond the valve ring either in native or prosthetic valve IE, giving rise to paravalvular regurgitation, valve dehiscence, septal and myocardial abscesses, fistulous tracts, pericarditis and conduction disturbances such as first degree AV block;
- a change in the quality of the audible prosthetic clicks can reflect valve obstruction by vegetation overgrowth. Because patients with prosthetic heart valves are always at risk for IE, the presence of fever or new prosthesis dysfunction at any time warrants consideration of the diagnosis.

Heart murmurs are heard in 80–85 per cent of patients with IE but may be difficult to detect and even absent in patients with tricuspid valve involvement. Careful auscultation in full inspiration is often useful in diagnosing right-sided murmurs. Septic pulmonary embolization from right-sided valvular IE (frequently seen in IV drug abusers) can give rise to shortness of breath, haemoptysis, pleuritic chest pain and pulmonary abscesses.

Poor prognostic factors include: increased age, infection of a prosthetic valve, patients with cardiac complications on admission, persistent sepsis, type of organism involved (*Staphylococcus*, fungal and nosocomial infections carry a higher risk compared to *Streptococcus viridans* infection) and the presence of associated diseases such as chronic renal disease, chronic liver disease, neoplasms and HIV.

Diagnosis and investigations

IE is largely a clinical diagnosis, based on history and clinical examination, that is confirmed with blood cultures and echocardiography. It is important to search for a portal of entry of infection, which may give a clue to the type of organism causing the infection. For instance, *Streptococcus viridans* infections frequently occur following dental procedures or poor oral hygiene, enterococcal infections occur after genitourinary and gastrointestinal procedures or in women after abortion or giving birth, and staphylococcal, Gram-negative bacterial, and fungal infections in drug abusers and after open heart surgery. Alternatively, the causative organism may be associated with an underlying condition, for instance *Streptococcus bovis* IE is frequently associated with colonic polyps and cancer. Most cases of procedure-related IE occur with a short incubation period of approximately 2 weeks or less following the procedure.

The variability in the clinical presentation of IE requires a diagnostic strategy that is sensitive for disease detection and specific for its exclusion. A strategy developed at the Duke University, USA, called the Duke Criteria, is currently recommended by the American College of Cardiology/American Heart Association (ACC/AHA) and has been adopted internationally to aid in the diagnosis of IE. A definite diagnosis of IE can be made either pathologically or clinically. A pathological diagnosis is made when pathological specimens from surgery or autopsy reveal positive histology or culture. A clinical diagnosis is made by determining the presence of major and/or minor criteria as seen in Box 8.1. A diagnosis of IE is made if there are two major or one major and three minor or five minor criteria.

Blood cultures are paramount for diagnosis and monitoring treatment. Three sets of cultures (aerobic and anaerobic) containing at least 10 mL blood should be taken from different sites, at different times (30–60 minute intervals), and before commencement of antibiotics. Blood cultures are negative in ≤5 per cent of patients with IE diagnosed by strict diagnostic criteria. Negative blood cultures may occur as a result of inadequate microbiological techniques, infection with highly fastidious bacteria or non-bacterial organisms, or prior administration of antibiotics before blood cultures were obtained. In patients who were given recent antibiotics and have a clinical syndrome of endocarditis, empirical antimicrobial therapy should be delayed or discontinued for up to 4 days, to allow blood cultures to be taken, provided the patient is not toxic, or has clinical or echocardiographic evidence of severe or progressive heart failure. Specialized microbiological techniques and culture media, prolonged incubation periods as well as serology (for organisms such as *Brucella*, *Legionella*, *Bartonella*, *Coxiella burnetii* or *Chlamydia* species)

Box 8.1 Definitions of terms used in the modified Duke criteria for the diagnosis of IE[a]

Major criteria
Positive blood culture for IE
Typical micro-organism consistent with IE from 2 separate blood cultures as noted below:

1 viridans streptococci, *Streptococcus bovis*, HACEK group, *Staphylococcus aureus* or
2 community-acquired enterococci in the absence of a primary focus, or

   Micro-organisms consistent with IE from persistently positive blood cultures defined as:

1 ≥2 positive cultures of blood samples drawn >12 hours apart or
2 all of 3 or a majority of ≥4 separate cultures of blood (with first and last sample drawn ≥1 hour apart).

Positive blood culture for *Coxiella burnetii* or antiphase 1 IgG antibody titre >1:800.

Evidence of endocardial involvement
Positive echocardiogram for IE defined as:

1 oscillating intracardiac mass on valve or supporting structures, in the path of regurgitant jets, or on implanted material in the absence of an alternative anatomical explanation, or
2 abscess, or
3 new partial dehiscence of prosthetic valve, or

   New valvular regurgitation (worsening or changing of pre-existing murmur not sufficient).

Note: TOE is recommended in patients with prosthetic valves who are rated as having at least possible IE by clinical criteria, or who have complicated IE such as paravalvular abscesses, etc.

Minor criteria

1 Predisposition: predisposing heart condition or intravenous drug use
2 Fever: temperature ≥38.0°C
3 Vascular phenomena: major arterial emboli, septic pulmonary infarcts, mycotic aneurysm, intracranial haemorrhage, conjunctival haemorrhages, and Janeway lesions
4 Immunological phenomena: glomerulonephritis, Osler's nodes, Roth spots, and rheumatoid factor
5 Microbiological evidence: positive blood culture but does not meet a major criterion as noted above or serological evidence of active infection with organism consistent with IE

[a] A diagnosis of IE is made if there are two major or one major and three minor or five minor criteria. Possible IE is suspected if there is one major and one minor criterion, or three minor criteria.
Adapted from Li *et al. Clin Infect Dis* 2000; **30**: 633–8.

may be needed to diagnose unusual organisms. Swabs should be taken from skin lesions, cannulation sites and the nasal cavity. Early and close liaison with the microbiology department is essential.

Echocardiography is not an appropriate screening test in the evaluation of patients with fever or a positive blood culture that is unlikely to reflect IE. Nevertheless, echocardiography should be performed in all patients suspected of having IE clinically. Transthoracic echocardiography is readily available, non-invasive and has a sensitivity of ≤60 per cent for vegetations >2 mm and a specificity of 98 per cent. In patients in whom IE or its complications are strongly suspected, a negative transthoracic echo will not definitely rule out IE and transoesophageal echocardiography (TOE) is recommended. TOE has a sensitivity of 76–100 per cent and a specificity of 94 per cent. It can diagnose vegetations ≤1 mm and is useful in evaluating and monitoring patients who develop complications and in patients with a suspected diagnosis of prosthetic valve endocarditis (compared to transthoracic echocardiography, TOE allows better visualization of prosthetic valves). Patients with native valves, in whom a clinical diagnosis of an abscess is suspected but not detected by TOE, should undergo magnetic resonance imaging (MRI). Patients with prosthetic valves can have MRI provided the prosthesis is MRI compatible. Most MRI departments have a list of MRI-compatible valve prostheses.

Haematological indices are frequently abnormal and include: a raised erythrocyte sedimentation rate (ESR), leucocytosis, normochromic normocytic anaemia, low serum iron and a low serum iron binding capacity. Findings of immune stimulation and ongoing inflammation include: a raised C-reactive protein (CRP), rheumatoid factor, hypocomplementaemia (decreased C3/C4) and cryoglobulinaemia. Urine analysis may show haematuria, red cell casts and proteinuria as a result of glomerular involvement. Although there may be no specific changes on the electrocardiogram (ECG), the development of PR interval prolongation may signify the presence of an aortic root or septal abscess. Chest x-ray may show signs of heart failure and pulmonary infiltrates from septic emboli.

It is important to recognize that the majority of symptoms, signs and laboratory investigations seen in IE are not specific and can also occur in other diseases such as connective tissue disorders, atrial myxoma, acute rheumatic fever and lymphomas.

Antimicrobial treatment and monitoring

If the diagnosis is suspected and cultures have been taken, then IV antibiotics should be commenced. Pending the results of microbiological specimens, a combination of a penicillin and an aminoglycoside (usually gentamicin) is still the most suitable first-line therapy for streptococcal and most enterococcal and staphylococcal endocarditis. The type of penicillin, the dose and the duration of treatment depend on the infecting organism and its *in vitro* antibiotic sensitivity, as determined by the minimum inhibitory concentration (MIC). The MIC is the lowest concentration of antibiotics that inhibits a given percentage of the organisms, (usually 90 per cent of a bacterial inoculum). Antimicrobial treatment regimens for adults as recommended by the Working Party of the British Society, for native and prosthetic valve endocarditis are as follows:

- *Streptococcus viridans* and *Streptococcus bovis*. If the organisms are fully sensitive to penicillin (MIC ≤ 0.1 mg/L), benzylpenicillin 7.2 g daily in six divided doses by IV bolus injections plus IV gentamicin 80 mg b.d. should be administered. A 2-week treatment regimen can be given provided all of the following conditions are met: absence of any cardiovascular complications such as heart failure, aortic insufficiency, conduction abnormalities, thromboembolic disease, native valve infection, vegetations less than 5 mm in diameter; and, a good clinical response within 7 days with the patient apyrexial, feeling well and with a normal appetite. If these conditions are not met or the penicillin sensitivity is reduced (MIC >0.1 mg/L) then continue the same regimen for a further 2 weeks. Patients who are allergic to penicillin should receive IV vancomycin 1 g b.d. (over at least 100 minutes). One-hour post-dose concentration should be about 30 mg/L with a trough concentration of 5–10 mg/L. Alternatively, IV teicoplanin 400 mg 12-hourly for three doses followed by a maintenance dose of 400 mg daily can be given. Vancomycin or teicoplanin is given for 4 weeks plus IV gentamicin 80 mg b.d. for 2 weeks. Gentamicin concentration should be determined at least twice weekly in patients with normal renal function. If renal function is abnormal, then it should be determined more often, such as every third dose. One-hour post-dose concentration should be 3–5 mg/L with a trough concentration of <1 mg/L.
- enterococci. For gentamicin-sensitive organisms (MIC < 100 mg/L), ampicillin or amoxicillin 12 g daily in 6 divided doses by IV bolus injection plus IV gentamicin 80 mg b.d. for 4 weeks should be administered. For gentamicin highly resistant organisms (MIC ≥ 2000 mg/L), the same doses of amoxicillin or ampicillin should be continued for a minimum of 6 weeks. Streptomycin can be given if the strain is sensitive. For patients allergic to penicillin, either vancomycin or teicoplanin plus gentamicin, at the previously mentioned doses and serum concentrations, should be given for 4 weeks.

- staphylococci. If staphylococci are isolated from blood cultures of a patient with suspected endocarditis, treatment should be started with vancomycin and gentamicin until the sensitivity is known when it can then be modified. With penicillin-sensitive organisms, benzylpenicillin 7.2 g daily in six divided doses for 4 weeks plus IV gentamicin 80–120 mg t.d.s. for 1 week should be administered. Close monitoring of renal function and serum concentration of gentamicin is essential. The 1-hour post-dose concentration should be between 5 and 10 mg/L with a trough concentration of <2 mg/L. Oral fusidic acid may be considered as an alternative to gentamicin for fusidic-acid-sensitive strains. For penicillin-resistant but methicillin-sensitive organisms, flucloxacillin 12 g daily in 6 divided doses for 4 weeks plus gentamicin 80–120 mg for 1 week should be administered. For penicillin- and methicillin-resistant organisms, IV vancomycin 1 g b.d. (optimize pre- and post-dose serum concentration as previously mentioned) for 4 weeks plus IV gentamicin 80–120 mg t.d.s. for 1 week should be administered. The latter regimen is also used in patients allergic to penicillin. While the duration of treatment rarely needs to be longer than 4 weeks for native valve infection, 4–6 weeks may be preferable for treating prosthetic valve endocarditis.

The antimicrobial therapy for patients with IE caused by unusual organisms is based upon very limited clinical experience and data from animal studies. A full discussion of the therapeutic regimens for most of these infections is beyond the scope of this chapter. In summary, infections caused by the HACEK group and Gram-negative organisms can be treated with IV ceftriaxone 2 g once daily or ampicillin 12 g daily in six divided doses, plus IV gentamicin 1 mg/kg t.d.s. for 4 weeks. *Pseudomonas* infections are treated with an antipseudomonal penicillin such as piperacillin 18 g/day plus high doses of tobramycin 5–8 mg/kg/day. Fungal infections (*Candida* and *Aspergillus* species) are treated with amphotericin B (250 μg/kg/day). Fungal infections are often difficult to cure with chemotherapy, and require cardiac surgery. *Coxiella burnetii* (Q fever) is treated with doxycycline plus either co-trimoxazole, rifampicin, ciprofloxacin or hydroxychloroquine. *Legionella* is treated with doxycycline or erythromycin.

Most patients with IE respond to appropriate antibiotic treatment within 72 hours, with a loss of fever and improvement in general wellbeing. If fever persists or recurs, then further blood cultures should be taken. The recurrence of fever during treatment does not necessarily indicate an unsatisfactory response to antibiotics, but may indicate a hypersensitivity reaction to drugs, phlebitis, an infection elsewhere or major immune activation (Table 8.2). Urine analysis should be done daily, ECGs

Table 8.2 Some causes of persistent or recurrent fever during treatment of infective endocarditis

Infection related
　　Intracardiac; Paravalvular/intracardiac abscesses
　　Extracardiac; Line infection, metastatic infection, mycotic aneurysms, spinal abscess, vertebral osteomyelitis, discitis, etc.
　　Antibiotic resistance; Seldom a cause especially if the infecting bacteria has been cultured and sensitivity determined

Antibiotic sensitivity
Can be associated with or without a rash, eosinophilia, and a rise in CRP in a patient who had been previously doing well

Major immune activation
Associated with progressive renal failure, vasculitis, emboli, etc.

Multiple organisms
Usually seen in intravenous drug abusers

Wrong diagnosis
　　Lymphoma, sarcoidosis, AIDS, tuberculosis, atrial myxoma, acute rheumatic fever, autoimmune disease such as SLE, etc.

should be obtained twice weekly and echocardiography weekly. A falling CRP and ESR are reassuring.

Anticoagulant therapy

Anticoagulant therapy has not been shown to prevent embolization in IE and may increase the risk of intracerebral haemorrhage. Patients with prosthetic valve endocarditis who are receiving chronic anticoagulant therapy should be allowed to cautiously continue. However, in the presence of cerebral emboli with haemorrhage, temporary discontinuation of anticoagulation is appropriate. In unstable patients or in those for whom surgery is planned, warfarin can be discontinued and replaced with unfractionated heparin, which can easily be reversed.

Complications and indications for surgery

Patients should be seen and examined daily for the development of complications, which have already been discussed. Among the complications of IE, heart failure has the greatest impact on prognosis. Heart failure is more frequently seen with aortic valve infections (29 per cent) than with mitral (20 per cent) or tricuspid (8 per cent) disease. The early onset of heart failure signifies the need for surgical intervention. Delaying surgery to the point of marked ventricular decompensation

Table 8.3 IE and Indications for Surgery

Absolute	Relative
• Moderate to severe congestive heart failure due to valve dysfunction	• Congestive heart failure resolved with medical therapy
• Refractory infection (persistent bacteraemia, relapse after optimal therapy – prosthetic valves) with lack of improvement after more than 1 week of antibiotics	• Relapse after optimal therapy (native valves)
• Fungal infection	• Culture-negative endocarditis with persistent unexplained fever
• Unstable valve prosthesis	• Vegetations >10 mm
• Significant dehiscence of prosthetic valves	• New regurgitation in an aortic prosthesis
• Perivalvular extension with septal and myocardial abscesses, fistulous tracts, atrioventricular block, rupture of sinus of Valsalva aneurysm, rupture of subaortic aneurysm	• Single systemic embolic event
• Large vegetation causing obstruction	

• Recurrent systemic emboli
  – several episodes
  – one episode with residual large vegetation	

can dramatically increase operative mortality, from 6–11 per cent for stable patients to 17–33 per cent for patients with heart failure. The incidence of reinfection of the newly implanted valve in patients with active IE has been estimated to be 2–3 per cent, which is far less than the operative mortality rate. Therefore, surgery should never be delayed to prolong preoperative antibiotic treatment. Other indicators for acute surgical intervention also include intracardiac abscesses and fistulous tracts, unstable valve prosthesis, persistent bacteraemia despite antimicrobial therapy, fungal infections, recurrent systemic embolization ($\geq$2 major embolic events) and large obstructive vegetations (>10 mm) (see Table 8.3). The duration of antibiotic therapy following surgery is dependent on the antibiotic sensitivity of the organism, the presence of paravalvular invasive infection and the culture status of the vegetation. Generally, in endocarditis caused by antibiotic-sensitive organisms with negative cultures of operative specimens, preoperative plus postoperative therapy should at least equal a full course of recommended therapy. Patients with positive intraoperative cultures and prosthetic valve endocarditis should receive a full course of antimicrobial therapy postoperatively.

Prevention

IE is a life-threatening disease and carries a high risk of morbidity and mortality despite modern antimicrobial and surgical treatment. It is therefore imperative, whenever possible, to try and prevent unnecessary infections, especially those in high risk groups. When determining which patients need antibiotic cover, it is important to consider the underlying cardiac condition (as some conditions are more often associated with endocarditis than others), the risk of bacteraemia associated with the particular procedure, and the likely organism that may propagate to give rise to IE. Generally, all patients with valvular lesions, congenital heart lesions and prosthetic valves should have antibiotic prophylaxis before dental procedures or surgical intervention involving the respiratory, gastrointestinal, urinary or genital tracts (Tables 8.4 and 8.5). The evidence supporting the use of antibiotic prophylaxis in patients who have undergone cardiac transplantation is limited. However, these patients are at risk of developing valvular dysfunction, particularly during episodes of rejection. Because of this, and the continuous use of immunosuppressive therapy, most transplant physicians consider these patients to be in the intermediate risk category and recommend prophylaxis.

Streptococcus viridans is the most common cause of endocarditis following dental or oral procedures, certain upper respiratory tract procedures, bronchoscopy with a rigid bronchoscope, surgical procedures that involve the respiratory mucosa, and oesophageal procedures. Patients (including those with prosthetic valves but excluding those with a history of IE) requiring these procedures under local or no anaesthesia, should receive amoxicillin 3 g, 1 hour before the procedure as a single dose. Patients allergic to penicillin or who have received more than a single dose of a penicillin in the previous month should receive clindamycin 600 mg, or clarithromycin 500 mg 1 hour before the procedure. Patients with a history of IE should receive IV amoxicillin and IV gentamicin (see below). For multistage procedures a maximum of two single doses of a penicillin may be given in a month; alternative drugs should be used for further treatment and the penicillin should not be used again for 3–4 months. If clindamycin is used, periodontal or multistage procedures should not be repeated at intervals of less than 2 weeks.

Patients (excluding those with prosthetic valves or a history of IE) requiring dental, oral, respiratory tract or oesophageal diagnostic procedures under general anaesthesia should receive IV amoxicillin 1 g

Table 8.4 Estimated risk of IE associated with pre-existing cardiac disorders

Relatively high risk[a]	Intermediate risk[a]	Very low or negligible risk[b]
• Prosthetic heart valves including bioprosthetic and homografts	• Mitral valve prolapse with regurgitation	• Mitral valve prolapse without regurgitation
• Previous IE	• Pure mitral stenosis	• Trivial valvular regurgitation on echocardiography without structural abnormality
• Cyanotic congenital heart disease	• Tricuspid valve disease	• Ostium secundum atrial septal defect
• Patent ductus arteriosus	• Pulmonary stenosis	• Arteriosclerotic plaques
• Aortic regurgitation and/or stenosis	• Hypertrophic obstructive cardiomyopathy	• Coronary artery disease
• Mitral stenosis and/or regurgitation	• Bicuspid aortic valve or calcific aortic sclerosis with minimal haemodynamic abnormality	• Cardiac pacemaker
• Ventricular septal defects	• Degenerative valvular disease in elderly patients	• Surgically repaired intracardiac lesions with minimal or no haemodynamic abnormality, more than 6 months after operation
• Coarctation of the aorta	• Surgically repaired intracardiac lesions with minimal or no haemodynamic abnormality, less than 6 months after operation	
	• Ostium primum atrial septal defect	
• Surgically repaired intracardiac lesions with persistent haemodynamic abnormality	• Heart transplant	

[a]Antibiotic prophylaxis should be given.
[b]Antibiotic prophylaxis is not recommended.
Adapted with permission, Copyright © 1995 Massachusetts Medical Society. All rights reserved. Durack DT. *N Engl J Med* 1995; **332**: 38–44.

Table 8.5 Recommendations for prophylaxis during various procedures that may cause bacteraemia

Prophylaxis recommended	Prophylaxis not recommended
• Dental procedures known to induce gingival or mucosal adjustment bleeding, including professional cleaning and scaling • Tonsillectomy or adenoidectomy • Surgery involving gastrointestinal or upper respiratory mucosa • Bronchoscopy with rigid bronchoscope • Sclerotherapy for oesophageal varices • Oesophageal dilatation • Gallbladder surgery • Cystoscopy, urethral dilatation • Urethral catheterization if urinary infection is present • Urinary tract surgery including prostatic surgery • Incision and drainage of infected tissue • Vaginal hysterectomy • Vaginal delivery complicated by infection	• Dental procedures not likely to cause bleeding, such as of orthodontic appliances and simple fillings above the gum line • Intraoral injection of local anaesthetic • Shedding of primary teeth • Oral radiographs • Tympanostomy tube insertion • Endocardial tube insertion • Bronchoscopy with flexible bronchoscope, with or without biopsy[a] • Cardiac catheterization • Cardiac pacemaker or ICD implantation • Transoesophageal echocardiography[a] • Gastrointestinal endoscopy, with or without biopsy[a] • Caesarean section • Vaginal delivery[a] • Vaginal hysterectomy[a] • In the absence of infection: urethral catheterization, uterine dilatation and curettage, uncomplicated vaginal delivery, therapeutic abortion, insertion or removal of intauterine device, sterilization procedures and laparoscopy • Circumcision

[a] In patients at higher than normal risk, such as those with previous endocarditis or prosthetic valves, prophylaxis may be chosen even for these procedures, according to clinical judgement.
Adapted with permission, Copyright © 1995 Massachusetts Medical Society. All rights reserved. Durack DT. *N Engl J Med* 1995; **332**: 38–44.

at induction, then oral amoxicillin 500 mg 6 hours later (if unable to swallow, the latter dose can be given IV). Alternatively, 3 g oral amoxicillin can be administered 4 hours before induction then 3 g oral amoxicillin soon after the procedure. Patients with prosthetic valves or a history of IE should receive IV amoxicillin 1 g plus IV gentamicin 120 mg at induction, then oral amoxicillin 500 mg 6 hours later. Patients who are allergic to penicillin or who have received more than a single dose of a penicillin in the previous month should receive IV vancomycin 1 g over at least 100 minutes then IV gentamicin 120 mg at induction or IV teicoplanin 400 mg plus gentamicin 120 mg at induction or IV clindamycin 300 mg over at least 10 minutes at induction. In addition, antiseptic mouthwashes such as chlorhexidine hydrochloride and povi-done-iodine applied immediately before dental procedures may reduce the incidence or magnitude of bacteraemia. Bacterial endocarditis that occurs following genitourinary, non-oesophageal gastrointestinal, and obstetric and gynaecological procedures is most often caused by *Enterococcus faecalis* and, rarely, Gram-negative organisms. Therefore, patients requiring these procedures are covered with broad-spectrum antibiotics using a combination of IV amoxicillin 1 g and IV gentamicin 120 mg just before the procedure, followed by amoxicillin 500 mg 6 hours later. Patients allergic to penicillin should be given either van-comycin or teicoplanin. If the urine is infected, then antibiotic prophy-laxis should also cover the infective organisms.

Key points

- IE is a challenging medical disease, which requires a high index of suspicion, and early diagnosis and treatment in order to be successfully managed.
- IE can involve multiple systems and can often present in a similar way to other conditions such as connective tissue disorders, atrial myxoma and lymphomas, and is therefore a great mimicker.
- Although the number of cases of IE related to rheumatic heart disease has decreased, this reduction has been balanced by an increased incidence of IE in IV drug abusers and the elderly.
- Advances in microbiology techniques and echocardiographic imaging (in particular, transoesophageal echocardiography) have improved the ability to diagnose IE.
- A multidisciplinary approach is necessary for decision-making during treatment, with consultation from cardiology, cardiotho-racic surgery and the microbiology departments.
- Patients with signs and symptoms of heat failure should be con-sidered for early surgical intervention.
- Administration of antibiotic prophylaxis is determined by the underlying cardiac condition as some conditions are more often associated with endocarditis than others, the risk of bacteraemia associated with the particular procedure, and the likely organism that may propagate to give rise to IE.

Key references

ACC/AHA Guidelines for the Management of Patients with Valvular Heart Disease. A report of the American College of Cardiology/American Heart Association Task Force on Practice Guidelines (Committee on Management of Patients With Valvular Heart Disease). *J Am Coll Cardiol* 1998; **32**: 1495–8.

Bayer AS, Bolger AF, Taubert KA *et al.* Diagnosis and management of infective endocarditis and its complications. *Circulation* 1998; **98**: 2936–48.

Dajani AS, Taubert KA, Wilson W *et al.* Prevention of bacterial endocarditis. Recommendations by the American Heart Association. *JAMA* 1997; **277**: 1794–801.

Durack DT. Prevention of infective endocarditis. *N Engl J Med* 1995; **332**: 38–44.

Durack DT, Lukes AS, Bright DK. New criteria for the diagnosis of infective endocarditis: utilization of specific echocardiographic findings. *Am J Med* 1994; **96**: 200–9.

Li JS, Sexton DJ, Mick N *et al.* Proposed modifications to the duke criteria for the diagnosis of infective endocarditis. *Clin Infect Dis* 2000; **30**: 633–8.

Mylonakis E, Calderwood SB. Infective endocarditis in adults. *N Engl J Med* 2001; **345**: 1318–30.

Oakley CM, Hall RJC. Endocarditis problems – patients being treated for endocarditis and not doing well. *Heart* 2001; **85**: 470–4.

Piper C, Korfer R, Horstotte D. Prosthetic valve endocarditis. *Heart* 2001; **85**: 590–3.

Working Party of the British Society for Antimicrobial Chemotherapy. Antibiotic treatment of streptococcal, enterococcal, and staphylococcal endocarditis. *Heart* 1998; **79**: 207–10.

Drug-related cardiac problems

Digoxin toxicity

Digoxin is commonly used in the treatment of chronic atrial fibrillation (AF) and heart failure. More than 10 per cent of patients receiving the drug have been found to have evidence of digoxin toxicity when admitted to hospital. Digoxin has a narrow therapeutic index (therapeutic concentration 1–2 ng/mL or 1.3–2.6 nmol/L) with toxicity occurring with serum concentrations >2.5 ng/mL. Serum concentration measurements must be taken at least 6 hours after the last dose. Toxicity can occur as a result of self-poisoning or more commonly from drug accumulation over a period of time, particularly in the elderly and patients with associated renal impairment. Drugs such as verapamil, captopril, quinine, quinidine, propafenone, flecainide, amiodarone, prazosin, spironolactone, tetracycline, erythromycin and carbenoxalone can also increase serum concentrations and predispose to toxicity. Agents causing hypokalemia or intracellular potassium deficiency, hypomagnesaemia, hypercalcaemia and hypothyroidism can increase myocardial sensitivity to digoxin, despite satisfactory therapeutic concentrations.

Clinical presentation

Clinical features of toxicity include: anorexia, nausea, vomiting, confusion, weakness, apathy, fits, paraesthesiae, visual disturbances (blurred vision, xanthopsia-yellow vision) and acute psychosis. Severe poisoning can cause hyperkalemia [by inhibiting the myocardial membrane adenosine triphosphate (ATP) pump] and metabolic acidosis.

Digoxin toxicity can cause various arrhythmias and conduction disturbances. These arrhythmias arise from several actions of the drug, which include:

- enhanced automaticity, which can give rise to various atrial and ventricular tachyarrhythmias;
- excess vagal stimulation, predisposing to sinus bradycardia and atrioventricular (AV) block;
- a direct depressive effect on nodal tissue, further contributing to bradyarrhythmias.

When these actions are present simultaneously, intoxication is highly likely and can cause the characteristic arrhythmia of atrial tachycardia with block. Usually an early sign of toxicity is the occurrence of ventricular ectopics, which can proceed to bigeminy, trigeminy or salvos. Other arrhythmias include junctional bradycardia, second or third degree AV block, ventricular tachycardia (VT) and ventricular fibrillation (VF). When concomitant medication elevates digoxin levels, the features of toxicity may depend on the agent added. For instance, quinidine predisposes to tachyarrhythmias, whereas verapamil and amiodarone predispose to bradycardia and AV block.

Management

If digoxin toxicity is suspected then the following steps should be taken:

- stop digoxin
- correct hypokalaemia if present
- check digoxin level
- monitor cardiac rhythm and correct any sustained haemodynamically significant arrhythmia that occurs.

Ventricular ectopics, first degree AV block and AF with a slow rate but haemodynamically stable, require no special therapy except drug withdrawal. For haemodynamically unstable bradyarrhythmias and AV block IV atropine 0.3–1 mg every 3–5 minutes to a total of 0.04 mg/kg body weight should be given. If there is no response, then temporary transvenous pacing should be instituted. Beta-adrenergic agonists, such as isoprenaline, should be avoided because of the risk of precipitating more severe arrhythmias. Supraventricular tachycardias can be treated with beta-blockers to control ventricular rate, but there is an increased risk of exacerbating AV conduction disturbances. Therefore, an ultra-short-acting beta-blocker, such as IV esmolol should be used initially (see Appendix A). Ventricular tachyarrhythmias can be treated with ligno-caine and magnesium. Magnesium possesses significant antiarrhythmic properties in the setting of digoxin toxicity. For more resistant arrhyth-mias phenytoin or preferably digoxin-specific antibodies (Digibind) should be used. Phenytoin should be given as 50–100 mg IV as a slow bolus, every 5 minutes, to a dose not exceeding 600 mg. Digibind can be strikingly effective for life-threatening digoxin intoxication, especially when there are severe ventricular arrhythmias or hyperkalemia. The reversal of toxicity is rapid with few adverse effects, apart from the devel-opment of hypokalaemia as the ATP pump activity is regained, and potas-sium is transferred from the extracellular to intracellular space. The use of Digibind should be considered when more than 10 mg digoxin has been ingested by previously healthy adults (4 mg in children), or when the steady-state serum concentration is greater than 10 ng/mL, or the serum potassium level is greater than 5 mmol/L in the setting of severe intoxica-tion. Digoxin levels may remain high, but most digoxin is bound to Fab fragments and is functionally inert. Therefore, measurement of digoxin levels is not reliable or useful following the administration of Digibind. Box 9.1 summarizes the calculation for the administration of Digibind.

Box 9.1 Digibind dosing regime

The dose of antibody depends on the body load of cardiac glycoside, which has to be counteracted. When requesting levels it is important to specify whether digoxin or digitoxin is to be measured as the assays differ.

To estimate the body load of digoxin or digitoxin from the amount ingested:

The body load of digoxin = the amount ingested × 0.80
or digitoxin   (mg)

To calculate the body load of digoxin or digitoxin from the plasma or serum digoxin or digitoxin concentration:

The estimated body load = plasma (serum) concentration of
(mg)   digoxin (ng/mL) × 0.0056
                          × body weight (kg)

The dose of antibody (Digibind) is about 60 times the body load (whether digoxin or digitoxin) rounded up to the nearest 40 mg. Sometimes up to 12 or 14 vials may be required.

The risk of provoking dangerous arrhythmias with electrical cardioversion is greatly increased in the presence of digoxin toxicity and is in proportion to the cardioversion energy used. Therefore, electrical cardioversion should only be used as a last resort for the treatment of life-threatening tachyarrhythmias, always starting at a low energy level (i.e. 10 J). Overdrive pacing can be considered in patients with refractory ventricular arrhythmias.

Haemodialysis is not useful because the drug has a large volume of distribution and is extensively tissue bound. For acute overdoses, oral activated charcoal should be given to adsorb any cardiac glycoside remaining in the gut and to interrupt the enterohepatic circulation.

Tricyclic antidepressant overdose

Tricyclic antidepressants (TCAs) result in significant mortality when taken in overdose due to the cardiovascular effects of hypotension, myocardial depression and arrhythmias. The onset of toxicity is rapid with the majority of deaths occurring within a few hours of presentation.

Clinical presentation

Early clinical features are due to the anticholinergic effects of the drug, and include dilated pupils, dry skin, dry mouth, decreased bowel sounds (ileus), urinary retention and tachycardia. Cardiovascular toxicity can rapidly ensue with the development of hypotension, arrhythmias and asystole. Toxicity results primarily from effects on the myocardial cell action potential, direct effects on vascular tone, and indirect effects mediated by the autonomic nervous system.

TCAs can inhibit the fast-acting sodium channel and are therefore similar to class 1A antiarrhythmic drugs. Consequently, TCAs can impair cardiac conduction and prolong repolarization. They also have a negative inotropic effect due to inhibition of calcium entry into myocytes. The inhibition of sodium channels is pH dependent with acidosis aggravating cardiotoxicity. Conversely, an increase in pH is protective by improving cardiac conduction and reducing negative inotropic effects. Impaired conduction in the His–Purkinje system slows propagation of the ventricular depolarization wave, and prolongs the QRS interval. QRS interval prolongation is the most distinctive feature of serious TCA overdose, and is usually seen as a non-specific conduction delay on the ECG. A QRS duration >120 ms is a good predictor of cardiac and neurological toxicity, whereas a QRS duration >160 ms is predictive of ventricular arrhythmias. Prolongation of repolarization causes an increase in QT interval, predisposing to *torsades de pointes*. Non-uniform slowing may cause unidirectional block and re-entry circuits to develop, analogous to ischaemic myocardium, resulting in VT; VT may be difficult to distinguish from sinus tachycardia in the presence of prolonged QRS and PR intervals (P waves may be obscured by the preceding T wave). A 12-lead echocardiogram (ECG) may help reveal P waves not visible on a rhythm strip. Ventricular fibrillation is usually a terminal rhythm that occurs as a complication of VT or hypotension. The PR interval in TCA overdose is often prolonged, but second or third degree AV block is rare. Sinus tachycardia is the most common rhythm disorder seen and is present in more than 50 per cent of patients.

Management

Management is generally supportive, with monitoring of respiration and cardiac rhythm. Owing to the possibility of rapid deterioration, gastric lavage, instillation of activated charcoal and intravenous access are recommended. A 12-lead ECG should be obtained because it may reveal QRS prolongation that is not evident on the single lead of a cardiac monitor. Any hypoxic, electrolyte or metabolic disturbances should be corrected. Even in the absence of acidosis, if there is cardiac involvement (QRS prolongation >140 ms, ventricular arrhythmias) or hypotension, 50 mmol sodium bicarbonate should be administered slowly (see Appendix A). Because marked alkalosis can be physiologically detrimental, arterial blood pH should not exceed 7.5–7.55. Treatment for sinus tachycardia is not generally needed. First degree AV block requires no treatment, second (type II) or third degree AV block should be managed with temporary transvenous pacing. Any unstable ventricular tachyarrhythmias should be treated with direct current cardioversion (DCC); if recurrent, lignocaine should be administered. The use of other antiarrhythmic agents is limited, and may aggravate cardiotoxicity. Overdrive pacing should be considered in patients with refractory ventricular arrhythmias. Seizures should be treated with diazepam, as other anticonvulsant agents such as phenytoin may aggravate hypotension and arrhythmias. If seizures cannot be adequately controlled, paralysis and ventilation are indicated to prevent further acidosis. A fluid challenge often corrects mild hypotension and may facilitate the management of more severe hypotension, which can be treated with inotropic and vasopressor agents. Noradrenaline is the vasopressor of choice, although dobutamine may be effective in the presence of a low cardiac output but adequate filling pressures.

Substance abuse

It is estimated that almost one in four people in developed countries have misused recreational drugs at some time during their life. Therefore, independent of clinical practice, most doctors will experience or have to manage the ill effects associated with recreational drug abuse at some point during their career. In addition to their effects on the central nervous system, many of these agents induce profound changes in the heart and circulation, which are responsible for a significant proportion of drug-related morbidity. The purpose of this section is to review the cardiovascular complications associated with some of the commonly misused recreational drugs.

Cocaine, crack, amphetamine and ecstasy

PHARMACOLOGY

These drugs all share similar adverse effects on the cardiovascular system, related predominantly to sympathetic nervous system activation. Cocaine and its free-base form, 'crack', act by inhibiting the noradrenaline re-uptake transporter in peripheral nerve terminals as well as stimulating central nervous system outflow. Circulating catecholamine concentrations can be elevated as much as fivefold in cocaine users. Cocaine has a short serum half-life of approximately 30–80 minutes, with 90 per cent being metabolized and excreted in the urine over a 2-week period. At high doses, cocaine can impair myocardial electrical conduction and contractility by blocking fast sodium and potassium channels and inhibiting calcium entry into myocytes. Amphetamine and its derivative ecstasy produce indirect sympathetic activation by releasing noradrenaline, dopamine and serotonin from central and autonomic nervous system terminals. The plasma half-life varies from as little as 5 hours to 20–30 hours depending on urine flow and pH (elimination is increased in acidic urine). Compared to cocaine, amphetamine lacks the local anaesthetic effect of inhibiting fast sodium channels.

CLINICAL EFFECTS

Sympathetic activation can lead to varying degrees of tachycardia, vasoconstriction, unpredictable blood pressure effects, and arrhythmias, depending on the dose taken and the presence or absence of coexisting cardiovascular disease. Although hypertension is common, hypotension as a result of paradoxical central sympathetic suppression, a late relative catecholamine-depleted state, or acute myocardial depression can occur. Myocardial depression may be caused by ischaemia, a direct toxic effect of the drug or mechanical complications (acute aortic rupture, tension pneumothorax, pneumopericardium, etc.).

Cocaine and amphetamine can cause myocardial ischaemia and infarction in patients with or without coronary artery disease. The mechanism of this is uncertain, but may be related to the elevated catecholamine concentrations, which result in an increase in myocardial oxygen demand, coronary artery spasm, platelet aggregation and thrombus formation. Cocaine can produce a procoagulant effect by decreasing concentrations of protein C and antithrombin III, and potentiating thromboxane production. Chronic use of cocaine and amphetamine can cause repetitive episodes of coronary spasm and paroxysms of hypertension, which may result in endothelial damage, coronary artery dissection, and acceleration of atherosclerosis. Creatine kinase concentrations can be elevated in both cocaine and amphetamine abusers, and are therefore not reliable indicators of myocardial injury. This elevation of creatinine kinase is probably due to rhabdomyolysis. Consequently, serum troponin concentrations, which are more sensitive and specific for the detection of myocardial necrosis, should be measured in patients in whom cocaine- or amphetamine-related myocardial infarction (MI) is suspected.

Paroxysmal increases in blood pressure can lead to aortic dissection or valvular damage that increases the risk of endocarditis affecting mainly left-sided heart valves. Endocarditis is often associated with unusual organisms such as *Candida*, *Pseudomonas*, or *Klebsiella*, and frequently has an aggressive clinical course with marked valvular destruction, abscess formation and a need for surgical intervention. Prolonged administration of cocaine or amphetamines can also lead to a dilated cardiomyopathy. Aetiological mechanisms include repeated episodes of subendocardial ischaemia and fibrosis, and myocyte necrosis produced by exposure to excessive catecholamine concentrations, infectious agents and heavy metal contaminants (manganese is present in some cocaine preparations). Non-cardiogenic pulmonary oedema and pulmonary hypertension can also occur with cocaine and amphetamine abuse. Although the precise underlying mechanism remains unknown, a direct toxic effect or alterations in central autonomic nervous system pulmonary vasculature regulation has been suggested.

The adverse cardiovascular changes and sympathetic stimulation associated with cocaine and amphetamine ingestion predispose to myocardial electrical instability, precipitating a wide and unpredictable range of supraventricular and ventricular tachyarrhythmias. The presence of fibrotic scars, myocardial ischaemia, and left ventricular hypertrophy can act as a substrate for re-entrant arrhythmias. The class 1 antiarrhythmic effect of cocaine can impair cardiac conduction causing prolongation of the PR, QRS complex and QT intervals, and a wide range of bradyarrhythmias including sinus arrest and higher degrees of AV block.

Some cocaine users practise drug inhalation in association with a forced Valsalva manoeuvre (the positive ventilatory pressure increases drug absorption and therefore can enhance the drug's effect), which can, rarely, be complicated by a pneumothorax or pneumopericardium. Sudden cardiovascular collapse may occur as a result of myocardial ischaemia and infarction, arrhythmias, acute heart failure, or mechanical complications.

MANAGEMENT

Similar principles apply to the management of the cardiovascular complications associated with these drugs. If the patient is agitated and anxious, then a benzodiazepine in sedative dosages should be administered as this can attenuate some of the cardiac and central nervous system toxicity.

In the treatment of hypertension, beta-blockers should be avoided, as they may be associated with unopposed alpha-mediated vasoconstriction leading to paradoxical increase in blood pressure, and coronary artery vasoconstriction. The combined alpha- and beta-blocker drug, labetalol, is theoretically preferable to selective beta-blockers. However, the alpha-blocking effect is relatively weak and therefore labetalol can also exacerbate hypertension. Hypertension can be safely managed with either an alpha-blocker such as phentolamine or with vasodilators such as hydralazine, nitrates and nitroprusside. When hypertensive crises lead to the mechanical complication of aortic dissection or acute valve rupture, emergency cardiothoracic surgery may be required.

Myocardial ischaemia should be treated initially with oxygen, aspirin, and benzodiazepine. If there is continuing ischaemia, then vasodilators such as nitrates or phentolamine should be administered in an attempt to reverse residual coronary artery spasm. Patients with persistent ST segment elevation should receive reperfusion with thrombolysis or percutaneous transluminal coronary angioplasty (PTCA).

The majority of arrhythmias are short-lived and terminate spontaneously, as the drug is metabolized and cardiac function returns to normal. Consequently, antiarrhythmic agents should be avoided if possible. Supraventricular or ventricular tachyarrhythmias associated with haemodynamic compromise require urgent DCC. Sustained haemodynamically tolerated supraventricular arrhythmias should be treated initially with adenosine. In the presence of a hyperadrenergic state, the short-lived inhibitory effect of adenosine may be a disadvantage, allow-ing reinduction of the arrhythmia. If adenosine is unsuccessful or the arrhythmia rapidly returns, the co-administration of an alpha-blocker in combination with a beta-blocker may be effective. In 'body packers' suffering from overdose after rupture of ingested packets of cocaine, calcium antagonist may accelerate gastrointestinal drug absorption by inducing splanchnic vasodilatation. Furthermore, cocaine has a com-plex and highly variable effect on myocyte calcium metabolism, pro-ducing an unpredictable clinical response to calcium antagonist. For these reasons, it may be preferable to avoid giving calcium antagonists to patients suspected of cocaine abuse. Bradyarrhythmias can be treated with atropine; however, its effect may be attenuated in the presence of a hyperadrenergic state, and temporary cardiac pacing may be necessary. In the presence of sustained ventricular tachyarrhythmias, lignocaine and magnesium have an acceptable safety and efficacy profile (despite theoretical concerns relating to the shared class 1 effects of cocaine and lignocaine). There is currently no reliable information on the safety and efficacy of other antiarrhythmic drugs.

In animal studies using cocaine, the administration of sodium bicar-bonate has been shown to have a beneficial effect on myocardial electrical stability. However, this may occur at the expense of inducing paradox-ical intracellular acidosis or adverse systemic metabolic changes, lead-ing to detrimental effects on myocardial function. Similarly, in severe cases of amphetamine overdose, a forced acid diuresis may be success-ful in rapidly clearing amphetamine from the blood and limiting tox-icity, but major detrimental metabolic changes in acid–base balance can be induced. These treatments require intensive and expert monitoring and should only be performed by clinicians with previous metabolic experience.

Lysergic acid diethylamide and psilocybin

PHARMACOLOGY

Lysergic acid diethylamide (LSD) and psilocybin (magic mushrooms) are commonly abused hallucinogenic agents that are structurally related, and have similar physiological, pharmacological, and clinical effects. LSD is about 100 times more potent than psilocybin. Street mushrooms are often adulterated with LSD. Both drugs are indole derivatives and chemically resemble serotonin. Their mechanisms of action are complex and include agonist, partial agonist and antagonist effects at various serotonin receptors. The clinical effects are related to their serotonergic, dopaminergic and adrenergic activities. LSD is metabolized by the liver and has a plasma half-life of 100 minutes.

CLINICAL EFFECTS

The adrenergic effects of these drugs are usually mild and do not produce the profound sympathetic storms seen with cocaine and amphetamine. Symptoms corresponding to general sympathetic arousal include dilated pupils, tachycardia, hypertension, and hyper-reflexia. Although cardiovascular complications are rarely serious, supraventricular tachyarrhythmias and MI have been reported. Changes in serotonin-induced platelet aggregation and sympathetically induced arterial vasospasm have been suggested as mechanisms contributing to these complications.

MANAGEMENT

Management is usually supportive, as the majority of symptoms resolve within 12 hours. Agitated patients should be sedated with a benzodiazepine. The use of neuroleptic agents should be avoided as they can intensify toxic effects. Supraventricular arrhythmias can be treated with adenosine or verapamil. Apart from benzodiazepines, pharmacological intervention for mild to moderate hypertension is usually not required. Treatment for dangerously high blood pressure and myocardial ischaemia should follow the same general principles described for cocaine and amphetamine.

Narcotic analgesics

PHARMACOLOGY

Morphine and its semi-synthetic analogue heroin are the most commonly misused narcotic analgesics. When used alone or in combination with other drugs, they account for over 40 per cent of drug-related deaths. Heroin is slowly metabolized to morphine, which has a plasma half-life of 2–3 hours.

CLINICAL EFFECTS

Narcotic agents act centrally on the vasomotor centre to increase parasympathetic and reduce sympathetic activity. This effect, combined with histamine release from mast cell degranulation, can result in bradycardia and hypotension. Drug-induced bradycardia along with enhanced automaticity can precipitate an increase in atrial and ventricular ectopic activity, AF, idioventricular rhythm, or potentially lethal ventricular tachyarrhythmias. Some narcotic drugs (such as the synthetic agent, dextropropoxyphene, a constituent of co-proxamol) have additional sodium channel blocking effects, which further contribute to their pro-arrhythmic potential.

Bacterial endocarditis, affecting mainly right-sided cardiac structures, is a well-known complication of intravenous narcotic drug abuse, sometimes associated with pulmonary abscesses. Heroin overdose can cause non-cardiogenic pulmonary oedema, the onset of which can be delayed for up to 24 hours after admission. As the oedema fluid has the same protein concentration as plasma, and the pulmonary capillary wedge pressure is normal, a disruption in alveolar-capillary membrane integrity has been suggested as a mechanistic cause.

MANAGEMENT

Initial management centres around ensuring an adequate airway, breathing and circulation. In the presence of respiratory depression, severe hypotension and bradycardia, administration of repeated boluses or an infusion of a narcotic receptor antagonist (Narcan) will be required, as detailed in Appendix A. In severe hypotension, the insertion of a pulmonary flow catheter may be needed to help guide fluid and inotropic administration, and avoid inappropriate administration of diuretics in patients with non-cardiogenic pulmonary oedema, which requires intensive ventilatory support.

There are no useful published data to guide selection of antiarrhythmic agents for the treatment of supraventricular and ventricular tachyarrhythmias. In the first instance, patients should be investigated, and hypoxic, metabolic and electrolyte deficits corrected. As the misused drug is rapidly metabolized, the majority of arrhythmias are short-lived, and it is therefore preferable to avoid the use of antiarrhythmic agents where possible to minimize the risk of pro-arrhythmic interactions. If treatment is needed for supraventricular arrhythmia, conventional agents such as adenosine, beta-blockers, verapamil and digoxin have been recommended. Ventricular arrhythmias should be managed along conventional lines. Persistent bradycardia may require atropine or temporary cardiac pacing.

The treatment of infective endocarditis follows the guidelines discussed in Chapter 8.

Volatile substance abuse

The abuse of volatile substances is an increasing problem amongst young male adolescents. The products used are legal, cheap, and easily available. Abusers generally employ deep breathing techniques with the volatile substances contained in a plastic bag or bottle, a crisp packet, or a soaked handkerchief, to maximize the inhaled concentration of the substance.

CLINICAL EFFECTS

Following inhalation, feelings of euphoria, excitement, and invulnerability can occur rapidly and are short-lived. Cardiac arrhythmias are presumed to be the main cause of death from volatile substance abuse. Volatile substances may induce supraventricular or ventricular tachyarrhythmias by sympathetic activation or by myocardial sensitization to circulating catecholamines. Some abusers directly spray the substances into the oral cavity, which can result in intense vagal stimulation and a reflex bradycardia. Profound bradycardia can evolve into asystole or secondary ventricular tachyarrhythmias. Some volatile compounds can reduce sino-atrial node automaticity, prolong the PR interval, and induce atrioventricular block. Myocardial ischaemia and infarction have been reported and are believed to be caused by a combination of coronary vasospasm, hypoxia or excessive sympathetic stimulation. Hypoxia can occur as a result of respiratory depression, aspiration, the placement of bags over the head and neck, intense laryngeal oedema and spasm, and the formation of carboxyhaemoglobin or methaemoglobin. Some volatile substances are structurally related to the agents used in general anaesthesia, and can therefore cause myocardial depression and hypotension. Chronic abuse can induce a poorly characterized cardiomyopathy.

MANAGEMENT

Patients should be managed in a calm non-threatening environment, with sedation if necessary. Hypoxia and chemical disturbances should be corrected to optimize myocardial electrical stability. Haemodynamically unstable tachyarrhythmias require prompt electrical cardioversion. Profound bradyarrhythmias may be treated cautiously with atropine or temporary cardiac pacing. Hypotension can be treated with intravenous fluids, guided by a pulmonary artery catheter, if necessary. Inotropic agents are best avoided, if possible, as they may induce refractory ventricular tachyarrhythmias in the electrically unstable myocardium. Calcium administration may help to reverse myocardial depression. In patients with sustained tachyarrhythmias, beta-blockers or amiodarone may help to combat sympathetic activation and are the antiarrhythmic drugs of choice. Cardiac ischaemia should be managed with oxygen, vasodilators, and reperfusion treatment. Cardiomyopathies are treated conventionally.

Cannabis

PHARMACOLOGY

Cannabis is the most widely consumed recreational drug. It has a plasma half-life of 20–30 hours and can be detected in the urine for several days in occasional users, and up to months in heavy users.

CLINICAL EFFECTS

Cannabis has a biphasic effect on the autonomic nervous system, depending on the dose absorbed. Low or moderate doses can increase sympathetic and reduce parasympathetic activity, producing a tachycardia and an increase in cardiac output. In contrast, higher doses inhibit sympathetic and increase parasympathetic activity, resulting in bradycardia and hypotension. Reversible ECG abnormalities affecting the P and T waves, and the ST segment have been reported. It is not clear whether these changes occur as a direct result of cannabis, independent of its effect on the heart rate.

Although supraventricular and ventricular ectopic activity can occur, life-threatening tachy- or bradyarrhythmias have never been reported. In patients with ischaemic heart disease, cannabis increases the frequency of anginal symptoms at low levels of exercise and may be a trigger for the onset of an acute MI. This is believed to occur as a result of drug-induced increase in blood pressure, heart rate and myocardial contractility, increasing myocardial oxygen demand.

MANAGEMENT

In the absence of major underlying structural heart disease, the autonomically mediated changes in heart rate and blood pressure are usually well tolerated and therefore no treatment is needed. Where necessary, hypotension usually responds to intravenous fluid administration. For significant bradycardia, atropine can be administered. Patients presenting with unstable angina or MI should be treated conventionally.

Key points

- The abuse of recreational drugs is common and it is inevitable that doctors will have to manage and treat their associated ill effects.
- Recreational drugs are complex and can induce profound changes in cardiovascular function, both acutely and chronically.

- Recreational drugs are often taken together, which can result in complex synergistic interactions with potentially detrimental effects.
- A high index of suspicion with early intervention and management is often the key to successful treatment.

Key references

Dick M, Curwin J, Tepper D. Digitalis intoxication recognition and management. *J Clin Pharmacol* 1991; **31**: 444–7.

Ghuran A, Nolan J. Recreational drug abuse; issues for the cardiologist. *Heart* 2000; **83**: 627–33.

Kelly RA, Smith TW. Recognition and management of digitalis toxicity. *Am J Cardiol* 1992; **69**: 108G–19G.

Lange RA, Hillis LD. Cardiovascular complications of cocaine use. *N Engl J Med* 2001; **345**: 351–8.

Mittleman MA, Lewis RA, Maclure M, Sherwood JB, Muller JE. Triggering myocardial infarction by marijuana. *Circulation* 2001; **103**: 2805–9.

Osterwalder JJ. Patients intoxicated with heroin or heroin mixtures: how long should they be monitored? *Eur J Emerg Med* 1995; **2**: 97–101.

Toxbase (National Poisons Information Service): http://www.spib.axl.co.uk

Williams DR, Cole SJ. Ventricular fibrillation following butane gas inhalation. *Resuscitation* 1998; **37**: 43–45.

Pericarditis

10

Background

Acute pericarditis is a clinical syndrome caused by inflammation of the pericardium and characterized by chest pain, a pericardial friction rub and electrocardiographic abnormalities. It is more common in adult males compared to women and young children. Common causes include idiopathic, viral, bacterial, uraemia, post-myocardial infarction, trauma and neoplasms (Table 10.1). The pericardial reaction can be purulent, haemorrhagic, fibrinous or serofibrinous. Complications may result in restriction of cardiac filling, either as a result of blood or fluid trapped in the pericardial sac (cardiac tamponade) or from thickening of the pericardium (constrictive pericarditis). These conditions may be prevented if diagnosis and management are undertaken early.

Clinical features

Pericarditis often presents with sharp chest pain, localized retrosternally or in the left precordial region, and exacerbated by breathing, coughing, moving or lying flat. The pain can radiate into the neck, jaw, arms, interscapular region, trapezius ridge, or upper abdomen and can therefore mimic acute myocardial infaction (MI) or an acute abdomen. The pain is relieved by sitting up and leaning forward. There may be a

Table 10.1 Causes of pericarditis

Infections	Viral: coxsackie B, echovirus, adenovirus, EBV, mumps, hepatitis B, HIV
	Bacterial: staphylococci, streptococci, rheumatic fever, *Haemophilus influenzae*, *Salmonella*, tuberculosis, *Neisseria meningitidis*, *Neisseria gonorrhoeae*, syphilis
	Fungal: histoplasmosis, *Candida*, aspergillosis
	Others: *Mycoplasma pneumoniae*, *Legionella*, psittacosis, rickettisae, actinomycosis, amoebiasis, *Echinococcus*, *Nocardia*, toxoplasmosis
Neoplasms	Primary, e.g. mesothelioma, angiosarcoma, teratoma, fibroma
	Secondary, e.g. lung, breast, leukaemia, lymphoma, melanoma, Kaposi's sarcoma, colon
Connective tissue disease	SLE, Still's disease, rheumatoid arthritis, systemic sclerosis, mixed connective tissue disease, polyarteritis nodosa
Drug-induced	Hydralazine, methyldopa, minoxidil, procainamide, dantrolene, daunorubicin, doxorubicin, cyclophosphamide and methysergide
Post-myocardial injury	Post-MI, Dressler's syndrome, trauma, post-pericardiotomy, pacemaker insertion, cardiac diagnostic procedures
Other	Idiopathic, uraemia, hypothyroidism, sarcoidosis, Behcet disease, radiation, oesophageal rupture

history of prodromal symptoms, which can include fever, malaise and myalgia. Dyspnoea may occur because of splinting of the chest from pain or because of significant accumulation of pericardial fluid (see cardiac tamponade chapter). A pericardial friction rub is often present and is best heard along the left sternal edge in the sitting up and bending forward position. The persistence of the rub throughout inspiration and expiration as well as when the breath is held can help distinguish a pericardial rub from a left-sided pleural rub. Large effusions can compress the base of the left lobe, causing an area of dullness and bronchial breath sounds just below the angle of the left scapula (Ewart's sign).

Diagnosis

General

Non-specific markers of inflammation including white cell count (WCC), erythrocyte sedimentation rate (ESR) and C-reactive protein (CRP) are usually raised. Cardiac enzymes may be elevated if the inflammation extends to the surface myocardium, and for this reason cardiac isoenzymes cannot always be used to differentiate between acute pericarditis and acute MI, particularly non-Q-wave infarction. Chest x-ray can be normal, or the heart shadow may be enlarged, suggesting the presence of a pericardial effusion. There may be pleural effusions but pulmonary congestion, if present, indicates associated myocarditis. Other specific haematological, biochemical and serological investigations are dependent on the suspected aetiology and include:

- urine and electrolytes (U&Es);
- antistreptolysin O titres, anti-Dnase B titre, throat swabs (acute rheumatic fever);
- blood cultures;
- acute and convalescent viral titres, monospot or Paul–Bunnell test (Epstein–Barr virus), cold agglutinins (mycoplasma), fungal precipitins;
- sputum, urine and faecal samples for microbiology;
- Mantoux test (tuberculosis);
- autoantibodies (lupus, rheumatoid arthritis, systemic sclerosis, etc.);
- thyroid function test.

Electrocardiogram (ECG)

ECG changes (Figure 10.1) can occur a few hours or days after the onset of pericardial pain and are characterized initially by concordant, concave ST segment elevation in all leads except leads aVR, V1 and sometimes V2 (these leads show reciprocal ST depression). The following evolutionary changes then occur: isoelectric ST segment with flattened T waves, isoelectric ST segment with T inversion and finally reversion of T waves to normal. These changes are different from cardiac ischaemia (Table 10.2). It should be emphasized that they may not follow an exact sequence and some patients may present with only ST elevation and a return to normal without T inversion. Alternatively, T inversion may be the first sign, since the acute process was missed. Pericardial effusion can produce low voltage QRS complexes and electrical alternans (see Chapter 12).

Echocardiography

Echocardiography is valuable for determining the presence and size of a pericardial effusion and monitoring progress if the effusion is drained or treated conservatively.

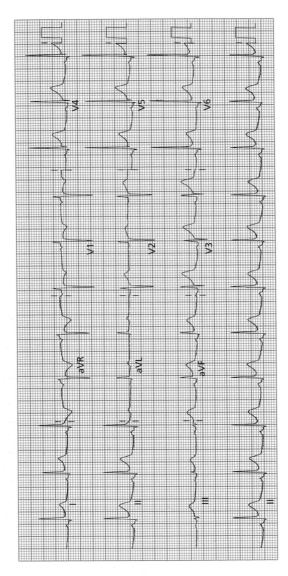

Figure 10.1 Electrocardiogram of a patient with an acute pericarditis.

Table 10.2 Progression of the electrocardiographic changes of pericarditis compared with myocardial infarction

Myocardial infarction	Pericarditis
Convex ST elevation	Concave ST elevation
ST elevation and T inversion	Isoelectric ST segment with T flattening and later T inversion
Loss of R-wave voltage and Q waves	Return to normal

Management

The first step is to establish whether the pericarditis is related to an underlying medical problem that requires specific therapy; for instance, uraemic pericarditis will require urgent dialysis. Non-specific therapy consists of bed rest until pain and fever have disappeared, and the administration of anti-inflammatory agents such as aspirin (600–900 mg every 4–6 hours), ibuprofen (200–400 mg every 6 hours) and indomethacin (25–50 mg every 6 hours). If these fail, a short course of prednisolone (e.g. 2 weeks) during the acute stage may be of benefit. Alternatively, colchicine has been shown to be effective for the treatment of both acute and chronic relapsing episodes. The dose for acute attacks is 1 mg followed by 0.5 mg every 2–3 hours to a maximum of 10 mg. The maintenance dose is 0.5 mg twice daily. With the exception of aspirin, anti-inflammatory drugs should be used cautiously in post-infarction pericarditis as they can affect scar formation and predispose to myocardial rupture. Antibiotics should be restricted to cases of purulent pericarditis and documented antibiotic-sensitive micro-organisms. Anticoagulants should be discontinued unless there is strong evidence for the development of thromboembolic complications. If anticoagulants must be continued, such as in patients with mechanical heart valves, intravenous heparin, which has a short half-life and whose action can easily be reversed with protamine sulphate, should be used. Patients should then be examined closely for the development of pericardial effusion. Aspiration of the fluid may be needed to confirm a diagnosis and/or to treat cardiac tamponade. Recurrent effusions may require the formation of a pericardial window, balloon pericardiotomy or the instillation of chemotherapeutic agents.

Acute idiopathic pericarditis is usually benign but may rapidly constrict or pursue a relapsing course before burning out. Late complications of pericarditis include pericardial fibrosis and/or calcification, resulting in constrictive pericarditis (particularly seen after episodes of tuberculous pericarditis), or a mixture of both effusive and constrictive pericardial disease.

Key points

- There are a number of causes of acute pericarditis but idiopathic, viral and post-MI pericarditis are the commonest.
- Occasionally the pain of pericarditis can mimic an acute abdomen or MI; however, in the majority of cases pericarditis has characteristic clinical and electrocardiographic features.
- Most symptoms resolve with rest and non-steroidal anti-inflammatory agents.
- With the exception of aspirin, non-steroidal anti-inflammatory drugs and steroids should be used cautiously in post-infarction pericarditis as they can affect scar formation and predispose to myocardial rupture.
- Late complications include effusive and/or constrictive pericardial disease.

Key references

Maisch B. Pericardial disease, with a focus on etiology, pathogenesis, pathophysiology, new diagnostic imaging methods, and treatment. *Curr Opin Cardiol* 1994; **9**: 379–88.

Oakley CM. Myocarditis, pericarditis and other pericardial disease. *Heart* 2000; **84**: 449–54.

Cardiac trauma

Background

In developed countries, cardiac trauma represents one of the leading causes of death in those under the age of 40 years. Young males are more likely to be affected than females. Road traffic accidents and physical violence are responsible for the majority of cases, although the incidence of iatrogenic causes as a result of intravascular and intracardiac catheterization as well as CPR is currently rising. Advances in initial resuscitation and surgical management mean more patients are surviving the initial insult.

Cardiac trauma is divided into penetrating and non-penetrating injuries. Both mechanisms can lead to myocardial rupture, contusion, laceration, pericardial insult, coronary injury, valvular damage, arrhythmias, and conduction abnormalities. Cardiac trauma is easily overlooked as attention is diverted to more obvious skeletal and multisystem injuries. As a result, haemodynamic instability can rapidly develop with devastating results. A high index of clinical suspicion with the early use of diagnostic techniques is essential and is often the key to successful management. It is important for physicians to have a good working knowledge of cardiac trauma to enable them to diagnose the occurrence of these conditions and manage the non-surgical components.

Non-penetrating cardiac trauma

Non-penetrating cardiac trauma usually occurs following the effects of direct external physical forces to the chest wall. The incidence of cardiac damage following this type of injury is estimated to be 10–16 per cent. Non-penetrating cardiac trauma most often is the result of road traffic accidents (as the heart is compressed between the steering wheel, and the sternum and spine) but can also occur as the result of falls, fights and sporting injuries. Box 11.1 summarizes the injuries that can develop as a consequence of non-penetrating cardiac trauma.

Cardiac contusion is considered the most common injury to the heart following blunt trauma; cardiac contusion usually produces no significant symptoms and can easily go unrecognized. Subepicardial and subendocardial petechiae, bruising, haematoma, lacerations and full-thickness myocardial damage, later followed by necrosis, fibrosis and aneurysm formation, can occur. The key symptom is precordial pain resembling that of myocardial infarction (MI) but unrelieved with nitrates. Other sites of chest trauma may confuse the clinical picture, but unlike injury to the thoracic wall, pain from cardiac contusion is not affected by breathing. There may be inappropriate tachycardia, gallop rhythm and a pericardial rub. The electrocardiogram (ECG) may show non-specific ST-T wave changes (Figure 11.1), findings of pericarditis,

---

Box 11.1 Consequences of non-penetrating cardiac trauma

Myocardium
- Contusion
- Laceration
- Rupture
  - Free wall
  - Septum
  - Valvular apparatus
- Aneurysm, pseudoaneurysm

Pericardial injury
- Laceration
- Pericarditis
- Post-pericardiotomy syndrome
- Constrictive pericarditis

Aortic dissection

Coronary artery injury
- Laceration
- Dissection
- Fistulae
- Rupture
- Thrombosis

Conduction disturbances
- Bundle branch block
- Bifascicular block
- Atrioventricular block
- Atrial arrhythmias
- Ventricular tachyarrhythmias
- Sinus node dysfunction

Commotio cordis (sudden cardiac death)

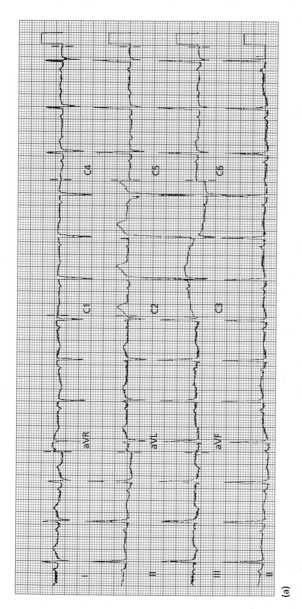

Figure 11.1(a) Non-penetrating cardiac injury sustained during a motor vehicular accident. Note the non-specific ST-T wave changes. There is T-wave inversion in lead III, and flattening in II and aVF. There was notching of the T wave in leads V3–V6. Reprinted with permission from Moriaty A. *Br J Cardiol* 1999; **6**: 578.

(a)

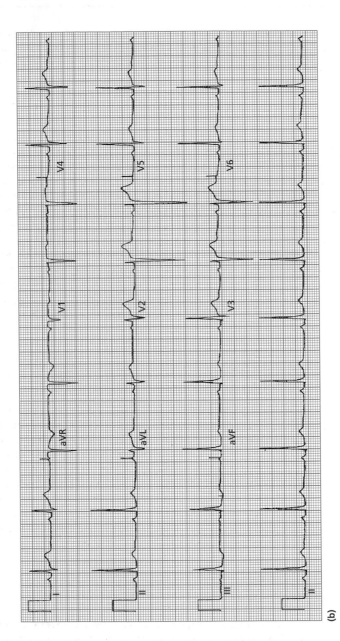

Figure 11.1(b) Repeat ECG a few weeks later demonstrates resolution of these changes. Reprinted with permission from Moriaty A. *Br J Cardiol* 1999; **6**: 578.

loss of R-wave amplitude and even pathological Q waves depending on the degree of injury. Localized injury to the conducting system can give rise to varying degrees of atrioventricular (AV) block, intraventricular conduction defects or bundle branch block. Supraventricular tachycardias, atrial fibrillation (AF), atrial and ventricular ectopics, ventricular tachycardia (VT) and ventricular fibrillation (VF) can also occur. Cardiac specific enzymes such as CK-MB isoenzyme, troponin T or troponin I can be used to make a diagnosis of cardiac contusion. Transthoracic echocardiography may show pericardial effusion, regional wall motion abnormalities, valve dysfunction and chamber enlargement. Up to 25 per cent of trauma patients cannot be satisfactorily imaged with transthoracic echocardiography and a transoesophageal echocardiogram (TOE) is a superior alternative. With the exception of anticoagulation and thrombolytic therapy, the treatment of cardiac contusion is similar to that of MI. Treatment is initially with bed rest and analgesia. Non-steroidal anti-inflammatory drugs are not advised as they can interfere with myocardial healing. In patients with marked ECG changes and/or significant thoracic or extrathoracic injuries, a period of intensive care unit monitoring for arrhythmias and congestive heart failure is indicated. Complete recovery usually occurs, as patients are often young with an otherwise healthy heart.

Cardiac rupture

Rupture of the free wall, interventricular septum, heart valves, papillary muscles, or chordae tendinae can occur acutely owing to the direct force of the injury or may be delayed up to 2 weeks resulting from necrosis. Rupture of the thoracic aorta commonly occurs at the aortic isthmus, just below the origin of the left subclavian artery. These complications are usually fatal. Patients may present with signs and symptoms of acute cardiac tamponade, severe congestive heart failure with a new murmur, or haemorrhagic shock. If indicated, pericardiocentesis may be life saving. Meticulous fluid resuscitation and early surgical intervention is the definitive treatment for most patients.

Pericardial injury

Trauma to the pericardium can range from contusion to laceration or rupture allowing herniation of the heart. Clinical findings include a pericardial friction rub and ST-T wave changes on the ECG characteristic of pericarditis. Complications such as haemopericardium and tamponade can occur. In the case of cardiac herniation, the heart becomes entrapped, there may be impaired filling and occasionally compression of the coronary arteries. There may be evidence of a displaced heart and pneumopericardium on a chest x-ray. The ECG can show a new shift in axis or bundle branch block. The only therapy for cardiac herniation is surgical repositioning. Uncomplicated pericarditis can be treated with non-steroidal anti-inflammatory agents. Recurrent pericardial effusions associated with pericardial pain, pyrexia and a friction rub can sometimes occur. It is similar to the post-pericardiotomy syndrome and is treated with non-steroidal anti-inflammatory agents. Constrictive pericarditis can occur as a late sequel and the treatment is total pericardiectomy.

Coronary artery injury

Coronary artery trauma includes laceration, dissection, rupture and fistulae formation. MI can occur if a coronary artery becomes occluded. A previously normal coronary artery may sustain disruption of the intima, subintimal haemorrhage and obstructive intraluminal thrombus formation on the injured arterial wall. Specific therapies such as systemic thrombolysis, intracoronary thrombolysis, percutaneous transluminal coronary angioplasty (PTCA) and stenting have been used successfully, but this depends on the timing of the diagnosis and associated injuries. Discussion with senior colleagues is essential.

Commotio cordis

Sudden death may occur in young sport participants when a small hard ball (such as a cricket ball) or other projectile (lacrosse ball, hockey puck, karate kick) strikes the victim in the precordium. This phenomenon is termed commotio cordis and affects children and adolescents 5–15 years of age without pre-existing heart disease. Characteristically, there is no structural damage to the thoracic cavity or heart. It is believed that an appropriately timed precordial blow, during the electrically vulnerable phase of ventricular repolarization, can induce a ventricular tachyarrhythmia and subsequently death. At present, early basic and advanced life support, and ensuring adequate chest protection are the only effective treatments against this phenomenon.

Penetrating cardiac trauma

Penetrating cardiac trauma is increasingly common with the majority being caused by gunshot and stab wounds, although shrapnel, fractured ribs, intracardiac diagnostic and therapeutic catheters can also produce penetrating cardiac injury. Penetrating wounds often result in laceration of the pericardium, as well as the underlying myocardium. One or more chambers, the interventricular and interatrial septa, valvular apparatus and coronary arteries may be involved. Box 11.2 summarizes the complications of penetrating cardiac trauma. In the case of stab wounds, the chamber most commonly involved is the right ventricle because of its anterior position, followed by the left ventricle, right atrium and the left atrium. Clinical presentation is dependent on the size of the wound and the location of the structures injured. If the pericardium remains open, blood can pass freely into the mediastinum and pleural space, causing haemorrhagic shock and massive haemothorax on chest x-ray. This is commonly seen in large or right ventricular wounds. However, if the pericardium does not permit free drainage because its opening has been obstructed by a blood clot, adjacent lung tissue or other structures, then blood accumulates within the pericardial space, causing cardiac tamponade. Under these circumstances, the chest x-ray will show a normal size cardiac silhouette, as the acute and rapid accumulation of fluid within the pericardial space does not allow distension of the pericardium. Echocardiography can be useful for diagnosing pericardial effusions, foreign bodies in the heart and intracardiac shunts.

Initial management includes securing the airway, establishing venous access and appropriately administered intravenous fluids and blood.

Box 11.2 Consequences of penetrating cardiac trauma

Myocardium
- Laceration
  - Free wall
  - Septum
  - Valvular apparatus
  - Coronary arteries

Pericardial injury
- Haemopericardium
- Pneumopericardium
- Pericarditis
- Post-pericardiotomy syndrome

Conduction disturbances
- Bundle branch block
- Bifascicular block
- Atrioventricular block
- Atrial arrhythmias
- Ventricular tachyarrhythmias

The offending object should remain *in situ* until exploratory surgery can be carried out. Patients who fail to respond to resuscitation and suddenly decompensate, should undergo immediate thoracotomy and repair of any treatable cardiac trauma. The incidence of late sequelae can be as high as 20 per cent and includes atrial and ventricular septal defects, tricuspid and mitral valve lacerations, and coronary injury. These complications may be missed on initial examination, only becoming apparent after a few days or weeks because of fibrous retraction of wound edges, resolution of oedema, ventricular enlargement and lysis of occluding clots. It is therefore essential that all post-cardiac trauma patients are closely monitored whilst in hospital and also in the outpatient clinic. Not surprisingly, penetrating cardiac injuries are usually immediately fatal, with the victim dying before reaching hospital.

Key points

- Cardiac trauma is a leading cause of death under the age of 40 years.
- It is divided into penetrating and non-penetrating injuries, which can both lead to myocardial rupture, contusion, laceration, pericardial insult, coronary injury, valvular damage, arrhythmias and conduction abnormalities.
- It is easily overlooked and should always be considered in anyone presenting with skeletal and multisystem injuries.
- A high index of clinical suspicion with the early use of diagnostic techniques is essential and is often the key to successful management.

Key references

Anderson DR. The diagnosis and management of non-penetrating cardiothoracic trauma. *Br J Clin Pract* 1993; **47**: 97–103.
Moriaty A. Myocardial contusion caused by seat belt. *Br J Cardiol* 1999; **6**: 577–9.
Westaby S, Odell JA. *Cardiothoracic Trauma.* London: Arnold, 1999.

Cardiac tamponade

Background

Cardiac tamponade is a clinical syndrome that occurs when blood or fluid fills the pericardial space, raising intrapericardial pressure and preventing ventricular diastolic filling. Consequently, there is a reduction in stroke volume and cardiac output with the development of shock. Tamponade is dependent on the rapidity of fluid accumulation and the distensibility of the pericardium and not the quantity of fluid. If accumulation is rapid, or if left ventricular function is compromised for other reasons, as little as 250 mL may be sufficient to produce tamponade. In contrast, it may take in excess of a litre of fluid to produce tamponade if it accumulates over a long period of time. Some common causes of cardiac tamponade are listed in Box 12.1.

Clinical presentation

Patients may present agitated or restless with hypotension, cold clammy peripheries, oliguria or anuria. In the setting of a more slowly developing cardiac tamponade, patients appear less ill and may present with anorexia, weakness and signs of biventricular failure such as shortness of breath, peripheral oedema and hepatomegaly. There may be an accompanying tachycardia, and the presence of pulsus paradoxus (an inspiratory decrease in amplitude of the palpated pulse or measured blood pressure) is supportive of the diagnosis. The jugular venous pressure (JVP) is markedly elevated with a prominent x descent and absent y descent. A positive Kussmaul's sign (an inspiratory increase in the JVP)

Box 12.1 Causes of cardiac tamponade

- Malignant disease
- Post-infective pericarditis
- Rupture of the free wall post myocardial infarction
- Uraemia
- Iatrogenic; post diagnostic (cardiac catheterization) or therapeutic procedures (pacemaker electrode insertion, angioplasty, etc.), anticoagulation
- Chest trauma
- Radiation
- Hypothyroidism
- Dissecting aortic aneurysm
- Post pericardiotomy syndrome
- Dressler's syndrome
- Connective tissue diseases e.g. rheumatoid arthritis, systemic lupus erythematosus, etc
- Idiopathic

---

is rare in cardiac tamponade. Its presence suggests that an organizing process and epicardial constriction is present, in addition to an effusion. The apex beat may not be palpable and the heart sounds are soft or even absent. There may be a pericardial friction rub.

In addition to a sinus tachycardia, the electrocardiogram (ECG) may show abnormalities of pericarditis, low voltage complexes and electrical alternans (alteration in QRS amplitude on a beat-to-beat basis as the heart continually alters its axis within the fluid-filled pericardial sac). The chest x-ray can show an enlarged globular heart shadow if the effusion is chronic or a normal cardiac silhouette if the tamponade develops acutely as seen during cardiac rupture or laceration. The lung fields are usually clear. Echocardiography is the definitive investigation, which will show the effusion and demonstrate the best approach for drainage. Echocardiography can also exclude other causes of systemic venous hypertension and arterial hypotension such as constrictive pericarditis, cardiac dysfunction, and right ventricular dysfunction.

Management

If haemodynamic compromise is present, intravenous fluids or inotropic agents can be administered to maintain haemodynamic support, whilst preparing the patients for pericardiocentesis (see below). Cardiac tamponade associated with cardiac trauma or aortic dissection requires immediate surgical intervention.

Pericardiocentesis

- Pericardial aspiration should ideally be performed with full x-ray screening, rhythm monitoring and resuscitation facilities readily available. Echocardiography can be used to guide pericardial aspiration as it allows visualization of the pericardial space, the myocardium and the aspiration needle. It can therefore give an indication of the best line of approach.
- The patient is placed at 30–45° to pool the pericardial fluid anteriorly and inferiorly. The patient is then connected to an ECG monitor.
- A long 18-gauge needle should be used. The V1 lead from an ECG machine is connected to the metal hub of the needle via a sterile alligator clip.
- Although several sites have been advocated for pericardiocentesis, the subxiphoid approach is preferred as it is extrapleural and avoids the coronary, pericardial and internal mammary arteries. The skin is cleaned and lignocaine 1 per cent infiltrated between the left side of the xiphisternum and the adjacent left costal margin, with the point directed towards the left shoulder, 45° to the skin.
- The needle is advanced whilst periodically aspirating and injecting small amounts of lignocaine. The needle is advanced until fluid is aspirated or until ST segment elevation and ventricular premature beats appear on the ECG, indicating that the needle has reached the epicardium. The right atrium is reached if there is PQ interval elevation. Alternatively, the injection of a few millilitres of contrast media can be used to determine if the needle is in the pericardial space, or within a cardiac chamber. If the contrast media swirls and is rapidly dispersed, then the needle is in a cardiac chamber. By contrast, the sluggish layering of contrast media inferiorly indicates that the needle is within the pericardial space. Failure of the bloody fluid to clot is further evidence that it is not from within the heart.
- The syringe is removed and a guidewire inserted under radiological or echocardiographic control. A pre-dilated pigtail drainage catheter is then inserted. Fluid can then be aspirated from the catheter. Removal of only 100 mL can produce a dramatic improvement in haemodynamic status. A connection is made to a collection bag if there is any possibility of fluid re-accumulating.

- Pericardial fluid should be sent for microbiology (microscopy, aerobic and anaerobic culture and sensitivity including requests for fungal and tuberculous investigations), biochemistry (protein and glucose) and cytology.
- The catheter is generally removed after 24–48 hours, to reduce the chance of infection.
- A post-procedure chest x-ray is obtained, to exclude a pneumothorax.

Rarely, following the removal of large amounts of pericardial fluid, sudden ventricular dilatation and acute pulmonary oedema may develop. This is probably related to a sudden increase in pulmonary venous blood flow, following the relief of pericardial compression in the presence of ventricular dysfunction.

Key points

- Cardiac tamponade is a clinical diagnosis caused by a critically increased volume of fluid within the pericardium, obstructing inflow of blood to the ventricles.
- Consider the diagnosis in any patient in a haemodynamically collapsed state, with a raised JVP, reduced heart sounds, low voltage complexes on the ECG and clear lung fields.
- Pericardiocentesis should only be done by those experienced in performing the procedure.

Key references

Callahan JA, Seward JB, Nishimura RA *et al*. Two dimensional echocardiographically guided pericardiocentesis: experience in 117 consecutive patients. *Am J Cardiol* 1985: **55**; 476–84.

Guberman B, Fowler NO, Engel PJ, Gueron M, Allen JM. Cardiac tamponde in medical patients. *Circulation* 1981: **64**; 633–40.

Krikorian JG, Hancock EW. Pericardiocentesis. *Am J Med* 1978: **65**; 808–14.

Appendices

Appendix A: intravenous cardiac drug regimens

Drug	Indication	Side effects	Pharmacokinetics	Dosing regimen	Comments/Cautions/Contraindications
Adenosine	Narrow complex tachycardia (SVT)	Flushing, chest pain, headache, dyspnoea, bronchospasm, nausea, excess sinus or AV node inhibition (bradycardia)	Half-life = 10–30 s. Rapidly metabolized by erythrocytes and endothelial cells	Initially 6 mg through a large central or peripheral vein followed by a flush of 10 mL saline. If necessary a further 3 doses each of 12 mg can be administered every 1–2 min	Dipyridamole potentiates the effect of adenosine. Methylxanthines (theophylline, caffeine) competitively antagonize the adenosine receptors and therefore higher doses may be needed. Contraindications: asthmatics, second or third degree AV block and sick sinus syndrome
Adrenaline	Cardiac arrest Anaphylaxis Inotropic support	Tachycardia, arrhythmias, hypertension, hypokalaemia, hyperglycaemia, headache, anxiety, tremor, sweating	Half-life = 2 min. β_1- and β_2-receptor agonist, high dose α-adrenergic vasoconstrictive effect	Cardiac arrest: IV = 1 mg (10 mL of 1:10 000 or 1 mL of 1:1000). Repeat as per resuscitation guidelines Anaphylaxis: initially, IM = 0.5 mg (0.5 mL of 1:1000). Repeat after 5 min in the absence of clinical improvement In some cases several doses may be needed. In severely ill patients with circulatory collapse, give IV 500 µg (5 mL of 1 in 10 000)	Cautions: ischaemic heart disease, diabetes mellitus, hyperthyroidism and hypertension

| Alteplase (Actilyse, rt-PA) | Acute myocardial infarction (MI) Pulmonary embolism (PE) | Minor and major haemorrhages, rash, nausea and vomiting | Half-life = 4 min. Metabolized by the liver. Binds to fibrin-associated plasminogen to form plasmin, which in turn breaks down fibrinogen and fibrin | MI: given as an accelerated regimen: IV 15 mg bolus, followed by 0.75 mg/kg (maximum 35 mg) over 30 min, then 0.5 mg/kg (maximum 35 mg) over 60 min. Give heparin IV 5000 U before commencing rt-PA, followed by 1000 U/h after completion of the rt-Pa infusion. Aim for an aPTT 50–75 s (1.5–2.5 times control)

PE: IV 10 mg over 1–2 min, followed by 90 mg over 2 h. Maximum 1.5 mg/kg in patients less than 65 kg. Give heparin as mentioned above | At present, few absolute contraindications as many are now relative, which needs interpreting within the clinical context. See section on thrombolysis, in Chapter 1 |

at a rate of 100 µg/min with ECG monitoring. Also give chlorpheniramine 10–20 mg IM/IV and hydrocortisone 100–500 mg IM/IV

Inotropic support: 5 mL of 1:1000 in 45 mL of 5% dextrose or normal saline (this gives a concentration of 100 µg/mL). The usual infusion dose ranges between 0.01 and 0.5 µg/kg/min. Higher infusion doses are acceptable depending on the clinical condition

Appendix A: (Contd)

Drug	Indication	Side effects	Pharmacokinetics	Dosing regimen	Comments/Cautions/ Contraindications
Amiodarone	Accessory pathway tachycardias, atrial fibrillation, atrial flutter Ventricular tachyarrhythmias Cardiac arrest (VF)	Pulmonary fibrosis, hyper/hypothyroidism, corneal microdeposits, skin photosensitivity and discoloration, pro-arrhythmic effect recorded though rare	Half-life = 25–110 days. Hepatic metabolism, lipid soluble with extensive distribution in the body	During cardiac arrest: VF/pulseless VT: amiodarone 300 mg, made up to 20 mL with 5% dextrose (can be given peripherally). A further dose of 150 mg may be given for recurrent or refractory VF/VT, followed by an infusion of 1 mg/min for 6 h and then 0.5 mg/min to a maximum daily dose of 2 g Stable tacharrhythmias: 150 mg diluted in 5% dextrose to a volume of 20 mL given over 10 min; this can be followed by a further dose of 150 mg if needed. Alternatively, a dose of 300 mg in 100 mL 5% dextrose over 1 h can be given. Follow with a continuous infusion of 900 mg in 5% dextrose over 24 h. Maximum recommended dose is 1.2 g in 24 h (European data sheet recommendation) although current resuscitation guidelines advocate that up to 2 g in 24 h can be used	Can increase digoxin and warfarin levels. Contraindications: sinus or AV node disease (unless fitted with a pacemaker) iodine sensitivity, pregnancy, breast feeding, thyroid dysfunction (relative) Administration via a central line is preferable to avoid thrombophlebitis during prolonged infusions. However, a large peripheral line is acceptable in the short term, until arrangements can be made to place a central line by skilled personnel

Drug	Indications	Side effects	Pharmacokinetics	Dose	Notes
Atenolol	Acute management of supraventricular tachyarrhythmias (including atrial fibrillation and atrial flutter) Myocardial infarction Angina Hypertension	Hypotension, bronchospasm, negative inotrope and chronotrope, peripheral ischaemia	Half-life = 6–9 h. Excreted by the kidney, not cardioselective, not lipid soluble	IV 2.5–10 mg at a rate of 1 mg/min	Acts synergistically with digoxin to control atrial fibrillation. Contraindications: heart rate less than 60 b.p.m., PR interval >0.24 s, second or third degree AV block, systolic arterial pressure less than 100 mmHg, uncontrolled heart failure (once stabilized an oral beta-blocker can be cautiously given), severe chronic obstructive pulmonary disease, history of asthma, severe peripheral vascular disease, Prinzmetal's angina, cocaine and amphetamine toxicity, and phaeochromocytoma
Atropine sulphate	Bradyarrhythmias Cardiac arrest (asystole)	Tachycardia, dry mouth, blurred vision (difficulties with visual accommodation), urinary retention, constipation	Rapidly cleared from the blood and is distributed throughout the body. Incompletely metabolized in the liver and excreted in the urine as unchanged drug and metabolite.	IV 0.3–1 mg every 3–5 min to a total of 3 mg or 0.04 mg/kg body weight During resuscitation IV 3 mg bolus (see resuscitation guidelines)	Contraindications: angle closure glaucoma (pupillary dilation can increase intraocular pressure), myasthenia gravis, prostatic enlargement (can precipitate urinary retention). These effects, however, are not

Appendix A: (Contd)

Drug	Indication	Side effects	Pharmacokinetics	Dosing regimen	Comments/Cautions/Contraindications
			A half-life of about 4 h has been reported		relevant to either the cardiac arrest situation or immediate post-resuscitation care
Calcium chloride 10% or calcium gluconate 10%	Hyperkalaemia Hypocalcaemia EMD arrest Calcium antagonist toxicity	Bradycardias and arrhythmias	Transient effects	IV 10 mL of the 10% solution. Give slowly	Avoid adding to solutions containing bicarbonate, phosphates or sulphates. Use separate IV access
Digoxin	Rate control atrial fibrillation, atrial flutter Heart failure	Anorexia, nausea, confusion, vomiting, visual disturbance. Arrhythmias including ventricular ectopy and bigeminy, paroxysmal atrial tachycardia with block, heart block,	Half-life = 36 h. Excreted mainly by the kidney. Peak effect may take up to 2 h. Therapeutic concentration 1–2 ng/mL (1.3–2.6 nmol/L). Toxic range	For atrial fibrillation, give 250–500 µg (orally) every 8 h for 24 h, then 125–250 µg daily thereafter. A loading dose is not necessarily required for use in mild heart failure. In renal impairment, reduce dose. For urgent loading, give IV 0.5–1 mg (diluted in 50 mL	Reduce dose in elderly and in renal failure. Hypokalaemia, hypomagnesaemia, hypercalcaemia, and hypothyroidism increase myocardial sensitivity to digoxin. Cautious administration in patients with hypertrophic obstructive

	idioventricular rhythm, ventricular tachycardia	>2.5 ng/mL	5% dextrose or normal saline) over at least 2 h	cardiomyopathy and atrial fibrillation. Contraindications: patients with Wolff–Parkinson–White syndrome, second or third degree AV block
Dobutamine	Inotropic support in cardiogenic shock	Tachycardias, arrhythmias, hypertension hypokalaemia	Half-life = 2.4 min. β_1-adrenergic receptor agonist, lesser β_2- and α-agonist effects	Given as an IV infusion between 2.5 and 20 μg/kg/min. Can be given peripherally. See Table A.1 for infusion rates according to body weight — Central haemodynamic monitoring recommended. Infusion can be given via a peripheral line

Table A.1 Dobutamine administration. Add 250 mg (5 mL of 50 mg/mL solution) in 45 mL 5% dextrose or normal saline (giving a concentration of 5000 mcg/mL). Commence infusion at 2.5 mcg/kg/min initially, slowly increasing to a maximum of 20 mcg/min. The following table gives infusion rates in mL/h for a solution of 5000 mcg/mL according to dose required and body weight

Dobutamine infusion rate (mcg/kg/min)	Body weight (kg)				
	50	60	70	80	90
2.5	1.5	1.8	2.1	2.4	2.7
5	3.0	3.6	4.2	4.8	5.4
10	6.0	7.2	8.4	9.6	10.8
15	9.0	10.8	12.6	15.4	16.2
20	12	14.4	16.8	19.2	21.6

Appendix A: *(Contd)*

Drug	Indication	Side effects	Pharmacokinetics	Dosing regimen	Comments/Cautions/ Contraindications
Dopamine	Low doses for renal perfusion Moderate doses for cardiac inotropic support High dose for peripheral vasoconstriction	As for dobutamine	Half-life = 5 min. Low doses stimulate renal dopamine receptors, therefore improving renal blood flow Moderate doses stimulate beta-(β_1) receptors High doses stimulate alpha-receptors	2.5 µg/kg/min for renal perfusion. 5–20 µg/kg/min for inotropic and vasoconstrictive effects. See Table A.2 for infusion rates according to body weight	Preferable to give via a central line, since extravasation from a peripheral line may cause severe ischaemic injury due to vasoconstriction

Table A.2 Dopamine administration. Add 400 mg (10 mL of 40 mg/mL solution) to 40 mL 5% dextrose to give a total volume of 50 mL, and a drug concentration of 8000 mcg/mL. The following table gives infusion rates in mL/h for a 8000 mcg/mL solution according to dose required and body weight

Dopamine infusion rate (mcg/kg/min)	Body weight (kg)					
	50	60	70	80	90
2.5	0.9	1.1	1.3	1.5	1.7
5	1.9	2.3	2.6	3.0	3.4
10	3.8	4.5	5.2	6.0	6.8
15	5.7	6.8	7.8	9.0	10.2
20	7.6	9.0	10.4	12.0	13.6

Appendix A: (Contd)

Drug	Indication	Side effects	Pharmacokinetics	Dosing regimen	Comments/Cautions/Contraindications
Esmolol	As for atenolol	As for atenolol, plus: confusion, thrombophlebitis and skin necrosis from extravasation	Half-life = 9 min. Selective β_1-receptor antagonist. Onset of action occurs within 2 min. Following discontinuation, full recovery from beta-blockade effects occur at 18–30 min. Metabolized by red blood cells	Give a loading dose of IV 500 µg/kg/min over 1 min before each titration step. Use titration steps of 50, 100, 150 and 200 µg/kg/min over 4 min each, stopping at the desired therapeutic effect	Can increase digoxin levels and prolong the action of suxamethonium. Interactions may occur with warfarin and intravenous morphine
Flecainide	Acute termination of atrial fibrillation. Accessory pathway tachycardias	QRS prolongation, pro-arrhythmic, negatively inotropic, dizziness, visual disturbances, ataxia, peripheral neuropathy, reversible increase in liver enzymes	Half-life = 13–19 h. Two-thirds hepatically metabolized, one-third excreted unchanged in the urine	IV 2 mg/kg or maximum 150 mg over 10–30 min. Maintenance infusion 1.5 mg/kg/h (in 5% dextrose or normal saline) for 1 h, subsequently reduced to 100–250 µg/kg/h for up to 24 h. Maximum cumulative dose in first 24 h = 600 mg	Contraindications: sick sinus syndrome, left ventricular dysfunction, intraventricular conduction delay or AV block, patients with a history of myocardial infarction. Can increase stimulation threshold in patients with permanent pacemakers, therefore use with caution. If QRS complex is prolonged by 20% from baseline, reduce dose or discontinue, until ECG returns to normal

Appendix A: (Contd)

Drug	Indication	Side effects	Pharmacokinetics	Dosing regimen	Comments/Cautions/ Contraindications
Glucagon	Reversal of beta-blockade side effects unresponsive to atropine	Nausea, vomiting, diarrhoea, hypokalaemia	Half-life = 5 min. Metabolized and cleared by the liver and kidney.	50–150 µg/kg in 5% dextrose as an IV bolus over at least 1 min. If the response is not maintained, a further bolus dose may be required (or an infusion in 5% dextrose of 1–5 mg/h)	
Glyceryl trinitrate (GTN)	Treatment of angina	Hypotension, headache, dizziness, flushing	Half-life = 1–4 min. Metabolized mainly by the liver and blood to dinitrates which are less potent	50 mg in 50 mL of solution as supplied by the manufacturer. Begin infusion at 10 µg/min (0.6 mL/h), increase by 10 µg/min every 15 min until a therapeutic effect is obtained. Maximum dose is 200 µg/min (12 mL/h)	Contraindications: hypotension, hypertropic obstructive cardiomyopathy, severe aortic or mitral stenosis, cardiac tamponade, constrictive pericarditis, cerebral haemorrhage. Tolerance with sustained blood levels
	Left ventricular failure and pulmonary oedema Hypertensive emergencies				

| Insulin | Hyperglycaemia | Hypoglycaemia, hypokalemia | 50 U of short-acting insulin (i.e. Actrapid or humulin S) in 50 mL normal saline. Administer according to sliding scale (see Table A.3) |

Table A.3 Short-acting insulin (Actrapid) sliding scale. Add 50 units of Actrapid in 50 mL normal saline to give a concentration of 1 unit/mL. The following table gives the infusion rates depending on the BMs

BM stick	Insulin infusion rate (units/h)
<5	0[a]
5.1–10	1
10.1–15	2
15.1–20	3
>20	6 (and urgent diabetologist review)

[a] Insulin-dependent diabetics require a maintenance infusion of 0.5 units/h.

Appendix A: (Contd)

Drug	Indication	Side effects	Pharmacokinetics	Dosing regimen	Comments/Cautions/ Contraindications
Isoprenaline	Heart block Severe bradycardia	Tachycardia, arrhythmias, hypotension, hypokalaemia, hyperglycaemia, headache, tremor sweating	Half-life = 2 min. Adrenergic agonist $\beta_1 > \beta_2$	5 mg in 500 mL 5% dextrose or saline (concentration of 10 μg/mL). Infuse at 0.5 mL/min (5 μg/min). Increase infusion rate to 1 mL/min to maintain adequate ventricular rate. The usual upper limit is 2 mL/min (20 μg/min). Isoprenaline is only used to maintain cardiac output until transvenous or transcutaneous pacing can be established	Caution: ischaemic heart disease, diabetes mellitus, and hyperthyroidism. Can increase infarct size and produce tachyarrhythmias
Isosorbide dinitrate	Angina Left ventricular failure	As for GTN	Half-life = 10 h. Metabolized by the liver to active mononitrate, excreted by the kidney	50 mg in 50 mL of solution as supplied by the manufacturer. Infuse between 2 and 10 mg/h. Maximum dose = 20 mg/h.	As for GTN
Labetalol	Blood pressure control in hypertensive emergencies or acute aortic dissection	As for atenolol	Half-life = 3–4 h. High lipid solubility, not cardioselective, alpha-blockade effect, metabolized by the liver	50 mg slow IV bolus over 1 min, repeat after 5 min if necessary (maximum 200 mg). For continuous infusion, commence infusion rate at 15 mg/h and every 30–60 min up to 160 mg/h. Discontinue infusion once blood pressure falls to desired level and initiate oral therapy	As for atenolol

Drug	Indication	Side effects	Pharmacokinetics	Dose	Comments
Lignocaine (lidocaine)	Ventricular tachycardia Ventricular fibrillation	CNS side effects including dizziness, paraesthesiae, drowsiness, confusion, convulsions and respiratory depression, hypotension, bradycardia	Effect of a single bolus lasts only a few minutes, then half-life = 2 h. Rapid hepatic metabolism	50 mg bolus over a few minutes. Can be repeated to a maximum of 200 mg. Follow up with an infusion of 4 mg/min for 30 min, then 2 mg/min for 2 h, then 1 mg/min over 24 h (500 mg in 500 mL 5% dextrose, gives a concentration of 1 mg/mL)	Reduce concentration in hepatic failure, congestive cardiac failure, following cardiac surgery and shock. Cimetidine and beta-blockers can increase blood levels
Magnesium sulphate	Persistent ventricular tachyarrhythmias Polymorphic ventricular tachycardia	Nausea, flushing, hypotension, confusion, weakness, loss of tendon reflexes, arrhythmias	Excreted by the kidney	Arrhythmias: 4 mL of 50% magnesium sulphate (8 mmol) in 100 mL of 5% dextrose or normal saline over 15–30 min IV. Repeat once if necessary. MI*: 8 mmol bolus over 20 min, followed by an infusion of 65–72 mmol over 24 h	Caution in renal failure and liver problems *The evidence to support the routine administration of intravenous magnesium in acute MI is controversial, and therefore the use of magnesium should be restricted to the treatment of recurrent ventricular arrhythmias
Metoprolol	As for atenolol	As for atenolol	Half-life = 3–7 h. Partially lipid soluble, cardioselective, metabolized by the liver	IV 2.5 mg over 2–4 min. May repeat every 5 min up to 15 mg	As for atenolol
Naloxone	To reverse respiratory	Nausea, vomiting, sweating,	Half-life = 60–90 min; therefore, short duration	Opioid overdose: 0.8–2 mg IV, repeated at intervals of 2–3 min	The duration of action of all opioids is often greater than

Appendix A: *(Contd)*

Drug	Indication	Side effects	Pharmacokinetics	Dosing regimen	Comments/Cautions/Contraindications
	depression induced by opioids	tachycardias. Can precipitate an acute withdrawal syndrome and non-cardiogenic pulmonary oedema in addicts	of action. Onset of action within 1–2 min following IV injection. Metabolized by the liver	to a maximum of 10 mg. For a continuous infusion: 2 mg diluted in 500 ml 5% dextrose or normal saline (4 mcg/ml), start infusion at 60% of the initial administered dose per hour	that of naloxone; therefore, additional doses (or a continuous IV infusion) of naloxone may be required. The patient should be closely observed following initial reversal. Use with caution in patients with pre-existing cardiovascular disease or in patients receiving cardiotoxic drugs, since arrhythmias (VT, VF, atrial fibrillation) can occur
Noradrenaline	To improve blood pressure in hypotensive patients by causing peripheral vasoconstriction	Hypertension, headache, palpitations, bradycardia, arrhythmias, peripheral ischaemia, extravasation can cause necrosis	Half-life = 3 min. Except in the heart, its action is predominantly on alpha-receptors	Comes as a strong sterile solution (2 mg/mL). Make up a concentration of 80 µg/mL by adding 4 mg (2 mL solution) to 48 mL of 5% dextrose, or 40 mg (20 mL solution) to 480 mL 5% dextrose (this gives a concentration of 80 µg/mL). Normal saline can also be used. The usual infusion dose ranges between 0.01 and 0.5 µg/kg/min.	Contraindications: hypertension, pregnancy, patients on monoamine oxidase inhibitors. Caution in patients with ischaemic heart disease

Drug	Indication	Side effects/Contraindications	Pharmacokinetics	Dose	Comments
Potassium chloride	Hypokalaemia	Arrhythmias		Add 20–60 mmol/L to 100 mL or 250 mL 5% dextrose or normal saline. Infuse at a rate no greater than 30 mmol/h. Concentrated solutions may be irritant and painful, therefore administer centrally if possible	Higher infusion doses are acceptable depending on the clinical condition. Contraindicated in renal failure
Propranolol	As for atenolol	As for atenolol	Half life = 1–6 h. Lipid soluble, non-cardioselective, metabolized by the liver	IV 0.5–1 mg every 5 min to a maximum of 0.15–0.2 mg/kg	As for atenolol
Reteplase (Rapilysin, r-PA)	Acute myocardial infarction (MI)	Minor and major haemorrhages, and hypersensitivity reactions (allergic reactions)	Half-life = 15 min. Recombinant plasminogen activator which catalyses the cleavage of endogenous plasminogen to generate plasmin. Primarily eliminated by the kidney and to a small extent by the liver; however, no dose change is required in renal or hepatic insufficiency	Reconstitute 10 U in 10 mL of the solvent provided (using the filter supplied). Give slowly over 2 min. Administer a further 10 U after 30 min. Give heparin IV 5000 U before commencing r-PA, followed by 1000 U/h after completion of the second r-PA bolus dose. Aim for an aPTT 50–75 s (1.5–2.5 times control)	At present, few absolute contraindications as many are now relative, which needs interpreting within the clinical context. See section on thrombolysis, in Chapter 1

Appendix A: (Contd)

Drug	Indication	Side effects	Pharmacokinetics	Dosing regimen	Comments/Cautions/ Contraindications
Sodium bicarbonate	Prolonged resuscitation (pH <7.1 or base excess ≤−10)	Tissue necrosis if extravasated. Administration can result in the generation of carbon dioxide, which diffuses rapidly into cells. This can result in a paradoxical intracellular acidosis; a negative inotropic effect on ischaemic myocardium; a high, osmotically active, sodium load to an already compromised circulation and brain; and a left shift in the oxygen dissociation curve, inhibiting release of oxygen to the tissues		50 mL of 8.4% (50 mmol/L) by slow intravenous injection	Do not administer via an endotracheal tube. Avoid adding to solutions containing calcium chloride or calcium gluconate. Use separate IV access
Sodium nitroprusside	Hypertensive crisis	Hypotension, cyanide or cyanate accumulation, lactic acidosis, hypoxia,	Rapid action, pre- and after load reduction. Effects wear off	Add 50 mg to 500 mL 5% dextrose (concentration 100 µg/mL). Prepare solution immediately prior to use, and	Caution in hypothyroidism, renal impairment, hyponatremia, IHD, impaired cerebral circulation.

Drug	Indications	Side effects	Pharmacology	Dose	Contraindications
		headache, dizziness, abdominal pain, perspiration, palpitations, phlebitis	1–10 min after discontinuation. Metabolized to thiocyanate and excreted by the kidney (2.7–7 days). Degraded by light	protect from light during administration. Initial dose (in a patient not already taking antihypertensive treatment): 0.3 μg/kg/min adjusting by increments of 0.5 μg/kg/min every 5 min to a range between 0.5 and 8 μg/kg/min. Maintain a blood pressure at 30–40% lower than pre-treatment diastolic BP. Fresh solution is required every 4 h, or earlier if it becomes discoloured. Duration of therapy should not exceed 72 h, and sudden withdrawal should be avoided. Terminate infusion over 15–30 min	Contraindications: severe hepatic impairment, severe vitamin B$_{12}$ deficiency. If infused for >24 h, give vitamin B$_{12}$ (hydroxycobalamin, 1 mg, IM). Check serum thiocyanate concentration (toxic level >100 μg/mL) or monitor blood gases for metabolic acidosis
Streptokinase	Acute myocardial infarction (MI). Pulmonary embolism (PE)	Minor and major haemorrhages, hypotension, rash, nausea and vomiting, allergic reactions including anaphylaxis, fever	Half-life = 30 min. Activates plasminogen	MI: 1.5 million units in 100 mL normal saline over 1 h. PE: 250 000 units over 30 min, then 100 000 units every hour for up to 12–72 h. Monitor clotting parameters	At present, few absolute contraindications as many are now relative, which needs interpreting within the clinical context. See section on thrombolysis, in Chapter 1
Tenecteplase (TNKase, TNK-tpa)	Acute myocardial infarction (MI)	Minor and major haemorrhages, and hypersensitivity reactions (allergic reactions)	Half-life 20–24 min. Derivative of human tissue plasminogen activator that binds to fibrin and converts plasminogen to plasminogen	Tenecteplase is dosed based on weight and is given as a single-bolus injection over 5 s (<60 kg = 30 mg, 60–69 kg = 35 mg, 70–79 kg = 40 mg, 80–89 kg = 45 mg, >90 kg = 50 mg).	This drug is not compatible with dextrose, and therefore should not be given in the same intravenous line. Lines containing dextrose should be flushed before and after

Appendix A: (Contd)

Drug	Indication	Side effects	Pharmacokinetics	Dosing regimen	Comments/Cautions/ Contraindications
			plasmin	Tenecteplase is supplied as a sterile, lyophilized powder in a 50 mg vial. Each 50 mg vial of tenecteplase is packaged with one 10 mL vial of sterile water for injection, for reconstitution. Give heparin, bolus of 4000 U and infusion of 800 U/h for patients ≤67 kg; 5000 U bolus and infusion of 1000 U/h for patients >67 kg). Continue infusion for at least 48 h. Aim for an aPTT: 50–75 s (1.5–2.5 times control)	administration. At present, few absolute contraindications as many are now relative, which needs interpreting within the clinical context. See section on thrombolysis, in Chapter 1
Verapamil	Narrow complex tachycardia (SVT) where adenosine is contraindicated or has failed	Sinus or AV nodal inhibition. Negatively inotropic.	Half-life = 4–6 h. Liver metabolized. Active metabolite norverapamil	5–10 mg over 2 min. A further 5 mg can be given after 5–10 min	Contraindications: hypotension, bradycardia, second and third degree AV block, sick sinus syndrome, cardiogenic shock, cardiac failure, broad complex tachycardia

Explanation of abbreviations can be found in the abbreviations list on pages ix–xi.

Appendix B: laboratory values and useful formulae

Laboratory values

Biochemistry	Reference range
Na	135–145 mmol/L
K	3.5–5 mmol/L
Cl	95–105 mmol/L
Mg	0.75–1.05 mmol/L
Urea	2.5–6.5 mmol/L
Creatinine	70–120 μmol/L
Creatinine clearance	80–140 mL/min
Bicarbonate	24–30 mmol/L
Fasting glucose	3.5–5.5 mmol/L
Calcium (total)	2.12–2.65 mmol/L
Calcium (ionized)	1.0–1.25 mmol/L
Phosphate	0.8–1.45 mmol/L
Alanine aminotransferase	5–35 iu/L
Alkaline phosphatase	30–300 iu/L (adults)
Bilirubin	3–17 μmol/L
Albumin	35–50 g/L
Aspartate transaminase (AST)	5–35 iu/L
Lactic dehydrogenase (LDH)	70–250 iu/L
Creatine kinase (CK)[a]	25–195 iu/L (males)
	25–170 iu/L (females)
CK-MB mass	< 5 μg/L
CK-MB mass:CK ratio	> 3 (MI likely)
Troponin T	< 0.05 μg/L
Troponin I[b]	< 0.1 μg/L
C reactive protein	< 8 mg/L
Free T4	9–22 pmol/L
TSH	0.5–5.7 mu/L

[a] CK values in healthy Afro-Caribbeans may be increased 2–3 times the quoted reference limit.
[b] Assay dependent, therefore check reference in laboratory.

Arterial blood gases	Reference range
pH	7.35–7.44
Pao_2	12–14.7 kPa[a]
$Paco_2$	4.7–6.0 kPa[a]
HCO_3	23–33 mmol/L
O_2 saturation	93–98%
H^+	36–44 mmol/L
Base excess	±2 mmol/L

[a] 7.6 mmHg = 1 kPa.

Haematology	Reference range
Hb	13.5–18.0 g/dL (males)
	11.5–16.0 g/dL (females)
WCC	$4–11 \times 10^9$/L
Neutrophils	$2–7.5 \times 10^9$/L
	40–75% WCC
Lymphocytes	$1.3–3.5 \times 10^9$/L
	20–45% WCC
Eosinophils	$0.04–0.44 \times 10^9$/L
	1–6% WCC
Basophils	$0–0.1 \times 10^9$/L
	0–1% WCC
ESR (increases with age)	<20 mm in 1 hour (rough guide)
	Age ÷ 2 (males)
	(Age + 10) ÷ 2 (females)
Platelets	$150–400 \times 10^9$/L
Prothrombin time	10–14 s
aPTT	35–45 s
Fibrinogen	2–4.5 g/L
FDPs	<10 mg/L

Haemodynamic pressures and parameters	Reference range
Left ventricle	
Systolic	100–140 mmHg
End diastolic	3–12 mmHg
Right ventricle	
Systolic	15–30 mmHg
End diastolic	2–8 mmHg
Aortic	
Systolic	100–140 mmHg
Diastolic	60–90 mmHg
Mean (diastolic + 1/3 pulse pressure)[a]	70–105 mmHg
Pulmonary artery	
Systolic	15–30 mmHg
Diastolic	4–12 mmHg
Mean	9–18 mmHg
Wedge (left atrium)	
Mean	2–12 mmHg
A wave	3–15 mmHg
V wave	2–10 mmHg
Right atrium	
Mean	2–8 mmHg
A wave	2–10 mmHg
V wave	2–10 mmHg
Systemic vascular resistance	700–1600 dynes s cm^{-5}
Total pulmonary resistance	100–300 dynes s cm^{-5}
Pulmonary vascular resistance	20–130 dynes s cm^{-5}
Cardiac output	5.5–9 L/min
Cardiac index	2.6–4.2 L/min/m^2

[a] Pulse pressure = difference between systolic and diastolic pressures.

Electrocardiography and echocardiography	Reference range
P wave width	<0.11 s (lead II)
P wave height	<2.5 mm (lead II)
PR interval	0.12–0.2 s
QRS duration	<0.12 s
QT interval[a]	0.44 s (males)
	0.46 s (female)
Aortic root	2–3.7 cm
Aortic cusp separation	1.5–2.6 cm
Left atrium	1.9–4 cm
Left ventricle diameter (end systole)	2.5–4.1 cm
Left ventricle diameter (end diastole)	3.5–5.6 cm
Left ventricular posterior wall thickness (end systole)	0.9–1.3 cm
Left ventricular posterior wall thickness (end diastole)	0.7–1.1 cm
Interventricular septal wall thickness (end systole)	0.9–1.8
Interventricular septal wall thickness (end diastole)	0.7–1.1 cm
Right ventricle (end diastole)	2.3 cm
Ratio of septum to posterior wall thickness	1.3 : 1
Fractional shortening	30–40%
Ejection fraction	50–85%

[a]When using drugs known to prolong the QT interval, discontinue or reduce dose if QT interval is greater than 0.5 s or increases by more than 60 ms from baseline.

Formulae

Bazett's formula (corrected QT interval) $= \dfrac{\text{QT interval (seconds)}}{\text{RR interval (seconds)}}$

LDL-cholesterol (Friedwald's equation) $= \dfrac{\text{Total cholesterol} - (\text{triglyceride} + \text{HDL-cholesterol})}{2.19}$

(Formula only valid for triglyceride concentrations < 4.5 mmol/L)

Cockroft and Gault formula for estimating creatinine clearance (mL/min) =

$$\dfrac{(140 - \text{age in years}) \times (\text{weight in kg})}{72 \times \text{serum creatinine in mg/dL}}$$

(for women multiply formula by 0.85; mg/dL = µmol/L ÷ 88.4)

$$\text{Body surface area} = \sqrt{\dfrac{\text{Height (cm)} \times \text{Weight (kg)}}{3600}}$$

Appendix C: useful web addresses

General	URL address	Content
American College of Cardiology	http://www.acc.org/	Clinical statements, ACC/AHA practice guidelines, links to other online cardiology journals, ECG of the month, echo of the month
BNF	http://www.bnf.org/	Drugs in the British National Formulary
British Cardiac Society	http://www.bcs.com/	BCS guidelines, meetings, education and training issues
Cardiac angiograms and coronary arteriograms	http://www.sbu.ac.uk/~dirt/museum/gs-sixth.html#11	Developed by South Bank University and contains normal and abnormal cardiac angiograms
Cardiac arrhythmias	http://www.arrhythmia.net/	Case histories, ECGs, diagnosis and management of various cardiac arrhythmias
Cardiology Compass	http://www.cardiologycompass.com/	A general overview of various cardiology procedures, image bank, links to other online cardiology journals and resources
Cardiosource	http://www.cardiosource.com/	Cardiology information resource service for cardiovascular news, clinical trials, Medline, trial acronyms, journal links (including the American College of Cardiology journal and Current Journal Review Scan), ACC/AHA practice guidelines
Doctors.net.uk	http://www.doctors.net.uk/	General medical information including cardiology forum, presentations, access to: *Clinical Medicine* by P Kumar and M Clark, *Clinical Biochemistry* by William Marshall, *Textbook of Paediatrics* by Forfar and Arneil, *Merck Manual of Diagnosis and Therapy*, NICE and SIGN guidelines, Clinical Risk Management, TRIP, *Hospital Medicine* journal and many more useful links
Doctorsworld.com	http://www.doctorsworld.com	General medical news, career information, a library which includes access to guidelines, formularies, clinical calculators, Merck's manual, *Gray's Anatomy*, *Emergency Medicine*, *Travel Medicine* and many more

ECG library	http://www.mrcppart1.co.uk/ecgs/ecghome.html	Excellent collection of ECGs
Electronic Medicines Compendium	http://emc.vhn.net	Provides free access to up-to-date, comprehensive and reliable information about prescription and over-the-counter medicines available in the UK
Emergency Medicine on the Web	http://www.ncemi.org/	Extensive resource on the management of acute medical emergencies. From e-medicine online textbooks, algorithms, calculators, nomograms, scoring systems, tables, key journals update, online dictionaries and many other useful links
European Society of Cardiology	http://www.escardio.org/	Educational resources, clinical statements, ESC guidelines
Freemedicaljournals.com	http://www.freemedicaljournals.com/	Access to available free online journals
Freewarepalm.com	http://freewarepalm.com/medical/medical.shtml	A collection of medical programmes such as drug databases, calculators, eponyms, biochemistry and haematology interpretation assistance, etc., that can be downloaded and used in a handheld computer
InCirculation.net	http://www.incirculation.net/frame.asp	Cardiology information resource service. Up to date reports on publications of interest, image bank, links to other useful websites and online journals
Lipidhealth	http://www.lipidhealth.org/	Issues regarding lipid management
Medicdirect.co.uk	http://www.dr.medicdirect.co.uk/main.ihtml	General medical resource centre. Lectures, slide library, leading edge articles, prescribers' journal online, drug update, career advice, clinical guidelines, clinical tools, clinical calculators and scores, patient information and videos
Medicines and Drug Information Centre	http://www.digri.demon.co.uk/drugs.htm	Excellent collection of links on drug information, from general prescribing to individual properties, adverse reactions and interactions

Appendix C: (Contd)

General	URL address	Content
Medscape.com	http://www.medscape.com/	General medical resource service with the option of receiving updates in chosen specialty
National library of medicine	http://www.nlm.nih.gov/	Medline, PubMed, Medline plus
North American Society for Pacing and Electrophysiology (NASPE)	http://www.naspe.org/	Heart rhythm information and resource for healthcare professionals and the public
QT Drugs.org	http://georgetowncert.org/qtdrugs.html	Drugs that prolong the QT interval
Resuscitation Council UK	http://www.resus.org.uk	A valuable resource for providing information on resuscitation, which is updated regularly. All new publications by the council are posted on the site together with details about forthcoming events, courses, membership and, when appropriate, important statements
The Cochrane Library	http://www.update-software.com/cochrane/cochrane-frame.html	Abstracts of Cochrane Reviews
The X-ray files	http://www.radiology.co.uk/xrayfile/xray/index.htm	A large collection of radiology cases, tutorials and useful links
Theheart.org	http://www.theheart.org/index.cfm	Cardiology information resource service. Up to date reports on publications of interest, image bank, links to other useful websites and online journals
Toxbase	http://www.spib.axl.co.uk/	Management of drug overdoses

Journals	URL address
Annals of Internal Medicine	http://www.annals.org/
British Medical Journal	http://www.bmj.com/
Chest	http://www.chestjournal.org/
Circulation	http://circ.ahajournals.org/
Clinical Cardiology	http://clinicalcardiology.org/
European Heart Journal	http://www.harcourt-international.com/journals/euhj/
Heart	http://heart.bmjjournals.com/
Hypertension	http://hyper.ahajournals.org/
Journal of Interesting EKGs	http://www.ekgreading.com/journal.htm
Journal of the American College of Cardiology	http://www.acc.org/
Journal of the American Medical Association	http://jama.ama-assn.org/
Lancet	http://www.thelancet.com/
New England Journal of Medicine	http://www.nejm.org/content/index.asp

Index

Page numbers in **bold** type refer to drug tables containing details of administration regimens